THE ROOTS OF HEALTH

Romy Fraser has been involved in Complementary and Alternative Medicine for over 20 years. In 1981 she established Neal's Yard Remedies, a company which provides natural remedies and high quality natural health products and promotes education and self-responsibility towards health. **Sandra Hill** is a Chinese medical practitioner and writer. Through 18 years of clinical experience, Sandra has discovered that self-awareness and self-responsibility are key to good health. Romy and Sandra met in the early 1990s when a group of like-minded alternative practitioners formed the 'Ecomedicine Group' to discuss the future of medicine. In 1998 they established a Foundation Course in Natural Medicines to provide a background to understanding alternative healing practices, and particularly the traditions of herbalism, homoeopathy, essential oils and flower remedies. Both the course and the ecomedicine group have been an invaluable background for the creation of this book.

Schumacher Briefing No. 7

THE ROOTS OF HEALTH

Realizing the Potential of Complementary Medicine

Romy Fraser and Sandra Hill

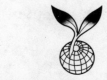

Published by Green Books
for The Schumacher Society

First published in 2001
by Green Books Ltd
Foxhole, Dartington, Totnes,
Devon TQ9 6EB
www.greenbooks.co.uk
greenbooks@gn.apc.org

for The Schumacher Society
The CREATE Centre, Smeaton Road,
Bristol BS1 6XN
www.schumacher.org.uk
schumacher@gn.apc.org

Cover design by Rick Lawrence

Printed by J. W. Arrowsmith Ltd
Bristol, UK

A catalogue record for this publication
is available from the British Library

ISBN 1 903998 05 0

Contents

Acknowledgements

Both Romy and Sandra would like to thank all members of the Ecomedicine Group and teachers and students of the Foundation Course in Natural Medicines. A particular thank you to Julian Barnard, Phil Beach, Peter Bruno, Patric Collin, Susan Curtis, Francesca Diebschlag, Peter Firebrace, Christopher Hedley, Pauline Hili, Tony Hurley, Irene Kohler, Hanelle Levine, Michael McIntyre, John Morgan, Neil Meikleham, Penelope Ody, Helen Stapleton, Beth Tyers and Ian Watson.

Introduction
and Summary

The 2001 Bristol Schumacher Lectures address three areas of major concern: for the health of society, the individual and the environment. Firstly, it is suggested that our lack of connection with nature and natural cycles may lay behind our spiritual malaise, which in turn will affect our physical health; secondly, our over-use and abuse of chemical substances in all areas of our lives, from the birth control pill and household cleansers to chemical fertilizers and the overuse of antibiotics in farming, is having a dramatic effect on our personal and environmental health. A move towards more natural methods of healing and the education particularly of teachers, health care professionals and children may provide hope for the future.

In his Schumacher Briefing *The Ecology of Health*, Robin Stott addresses the current state of medical practice within the UK and discusses many of the political and social implications of health and health care. His suggestions involve the changing from within of the present structure towards a more ecofriendly, patient-based human scale and holistic form of health care. We would like to suggest that change within the system will come from both within and without. It is by patient pressure that change will ultimately take place. The public is demanding a change to health care, and is showing its approval of complementary and alternative practices by visiting its practitioners in ever increasing numbers. In this Briefing we put forward some of the ways in which complementary and alternative medicine can contribute to the future of health.

Chapter One

The Roots of Health

'La Santé, c'est le luxe de pouvoir tomber malade et de s'en relever'
—George Ganghiler
(Health is the luxury of being able to fall ill and to recover.)

"I have an earache!"

2000 BC   "Here, eat this root."

1000AD   "This root is heathen. Here, say this prayer."

1800AD   "That Prayer is superstition. Here drink this potion."

1900 AD   "That potion is snake oil. Here, take this pill."

1950 AD   "That pill is ineffective. Here, take this antibiotic."

2000 AD   "That antibiotic is artificial. Here, eat this root."

The advancements of modern biomedicine have provided a sophisticated but somewhat mechanistic approach to health. It is an approach which is able to function well in emergencies, but which has fallen down in the more basic areas of maintaining and creating health. Dazzled by the progress of science, we have lost touch with the simple remedies and body wisdom that were once a part of every household. Throughout this briefing, we would like to suggest that Complementary and Alternative Medicine (CAM) has a central part to play in the future of health care. Both by looking into the past and reclaiming some of the more traditional views of health and disease, and by looking into the future and encouraging the application of appropriate scientific research into the body and its energy systems, we can begin to re-introduce balance into a system which is spiralling rapidly out of control. We would like to question the usual assumption that CAM is unscientific by suggesting that there are many ways to measure success and failure, and that possibly a qualitative rather than a quantitative approach is needed to evaluate health.

Over the past twenty years alternative and complementary medicines have steadily grown in popularity. Patient demand has created a place for complementary medicine within many mainstream practices. This popularity is not simply a matter of safer treatment without side effects, or even the personal time spent in consultation. Many alternative therapies are able to offer a different view of health, to put symptoms in perspective, to provide a framework in which the patient is able to understand the disease process and to become a part of the cure.

Many of the disciplines within CAM have their roots in the traditions of the past, and have embraced a philosophy of health which informs their practice. Most traditional systems of healing share a common philosophical ground based on an understanding of nature and of natural cycles. They provide a world view of mankind living in harmony with nature and in contact with a world of spirit. The human body is seen as an extension of the earth, our spirit as an expression of heaven or the divine. In many traditional systems, the earth is called the mother, the sky or the spirit, the father. In Chinese medicine these polar opposites are referred to as *yin* and *yang*, essence and spirit, in the Ayurvedic traditions of India as matter and consciousness, where *Purusha*, the unmanifest consciousness, unites with *prakriti*, the material universe, to create life. In each case the two are held in an embrace which is the very essence of life. Similarly both Northern and Southern American traditions maintain that all nature is imbued with spirit. These traditional world views engender a respect for life and a respect for nature.

The roots of medicine lie in a distant time when mankind lived close to the earth and depended on an understanding of nature and climate for survival. There was an understanding that the laws of nature are reflected in the laws which govern our bodies and therefore our health and wellbeing. The Western herbal tradition, for example, grew out of the Greek system of the four elements, the four temperaments and the four humours, which is based on observation of the natural world and the ways in which we respond to it. It assigns the attributes of hot, cold, moist and dry to each element and its appropriate season, but also recognizes related disease patterns and both constitutional and personality types, developing a complex system of resonances, in which a particular 'type' may be likely to respond to a particular medicine. In many cultures, diseases are described as cold or hot, moist or dry, and herbal remedies may be prescribed on the basis of their warming or cooling, moistening or drying properties. Herbs are also classified by their taste, which is a sign of their effects within the body. Herbs will be described for example as bitter, sweet, astringent. A similar system underlies that of Chinese medicine, where the five elements or five phases (*wu xing*) are drawn from observation of the energetic changes throughout the four seasons. Earth, at the centre, creates the fifth element, and supports each phase of change and transformation. In the Chinese system, each climate and taste is seen to have a particular resonance with an organ system. Native North American traditions hold similar views, attributing specific qualities to the seasons and directions.

In Chinese medicine, disease is classified by eight factors; hot and cold, internal and external, full and empty, *yin* and *yang*. A Chinese doctor's diagnosis will often begin by differentiating between these pairs of opposite qualities. Similarly, in Mayan culture disease is differentiated as hot or cold, ill health often referred to as cold entering the body, and death being the ultimate cold state. Not surprisingly, a large percentage of Mayan herbs are considered as warming, and are used to treat the various cold conditions. Similarly, the earliest and still most influential of the Chinese herbal texts is the *Shan Han Lun*, the compendium of 'cold diseases', compiled during the first century AD, and the most valued of herbal tonics are those that warm and strengthen. The Mayans also recognize 'hot diseases',

which refer to local conditions such as local infections, skin erup-
tions and fevers. It was not until the 10th century that Chinese
medicine recognized 'hot diseases', and the *Wen Bing Lun*, or compendium of hot diseases, lays down strategies for the herbal treatment of fevers. It is interesting to note that this discovery of hot diseases within Chinese medicine arrived at a time when settlements
began to move towards larger communities and more urban popu-
lations. Fevers and epidemics became a problem for the first time,
and new strategies of healing were required. It is also a reminder of
how medicine always reflects its cultural and historical context.
Traditional medical practices tend to be regional, and specific remedies will often reflect the specific needs and requirements of a local
environment and climatic region.

This acknowledgement of the cycles of nature, of the seasons and
the climates in traditional healing systems, is also reflected in an
understanding of the natural cycles of life. A similarity will be seen
in the practices which grew up in the Northern hemisphere, where
the spring represents birth and beginnings, the summer fruition and
growth, the autumn harvesting and decline, the winter death and
renewal. Although different in their detail, these cyclical cosmological maps are common to the Galenic, Chinese and Native North
American cultures. The observation of nature teaches that the seed
within the earth in the depths of winter is the beginning of a new
life in the spring; that decline naturally follows growth and fruition.
Traditional healing systems relate the rhythms of the body to the
rhythms of nature: an understanding of nature automatically
assumes an understanding of health. They also stress the importance of balance. Whether a balance of heat and cold, growth and
decline, or between the individual and the environment, balance is
seen as the key to good health. Within the Galenic tradition, the
melancholic temperament will tend to be chilly and pessimistic, and
could be prescribed warming herbs and vigorous exercise in order
to bring balance to the system. To the Chinese, anger may be a
manifestation of an unbalanced liver energy; it will be interpreted as
a lack of 'free flow' of energy reflected in an inability to relate well

with others. The blockage to this free flow will be discovered, and addressed with herbs, acupuncture, massage, diet, exercise or whatever may be appropriate.

According to Native American Cree healer Lea Bill:

> The systems within the world of plants, animals, trees, rocks and the atmosphere all contribute to the overall understanding of life processes and the principles of cause and effect. The imbalance in one system ultimately affects the other. The natural world celebrates our healing as it means greater opportunity for increased balance and biodiversity. Both systems strive for balance in their own manner, whether it is of mind body, spirit or emotion. Humanity and the environment are stewards of each other.[1]

Spirits and shamans

Our attitudes towards these traditional healing systems has been changing throughout the last century. The original confrontation between Western orthodox science and what it saw as a variety of apparently magical and most definitely heathen medical practices was one of total rejection. In recent decades, the field of medical anthropology has provided vital information about many traditional and tribal healing practices. In their article 'A General Overview of Mayan Ethnomedicine', E. A. and B. Berlin point out that in the preoccupation with the cosmological or magical aspects of Mayan healing, it has often been dismissed as superstition.[2] The Mayans' assumed lack of knowledge of human anatomy and physiology was considered to prove its lack of scientific basis. But the Berlins' research has shown their understanding of the medicinal qualities of plants to be extremely complex and their diagnosis accurate:

> In this sense, highland Maya traditional medicine is an ethnoscientific system of traditional knowledge based on astute and accurate observation that could only have been elaborated on the basis of many years of explicit experimentation with the effects of herbal remedies on bodily functions.[3]

The ethnobotanical knowledge of tribal peoples is now being recognized, and possibly already exploited by the pharmaceutical companies hungry for more medicinal patents. But we still tend to dismiss as magic and hocus pocus some of the more ritualistic healing
practices. The Berlins' work suggests that a case of diarrhoea, for
example, may be treated successfully with herbs either by self-medication or with the help of a local herbalist. But if the illness does not
respond to the usual treatment, the advice of a healer or shaman
may be sought, as the illness may be a case of 'spirit possession',
particularly involving an encounter with an ancestral ghost. Herbal
remedies may still be used in treatment but these will be accompa-
nied by prayers, healing rituals, ceremonial chants etc. Tibetan
medicine recognizes four categories of illness, the first can be
treated by adjusting behaviour and diet, the second needs to be
treated by medicines, while the third is due to 'evil spirits' and must
be referred to the lamas for prayers and exorcism before any other
treatment will be effective. The fourth category covers disorders
which result from actions in a previous lifetime. This is the most serious category of disease, and may be fatal. In the Tibetan tradition,
once this diagnosis has been made the patient may be encouraged
to devote their life to spiritual practice. Even in modern day Japan,
if a disease is not cured by the usual means, and especially if it
becomes progressively worse despite treatment, a priest may be
sought to look into the spiritual dimensions of the illness. Before we
dismiss these more obscure and occult healing practices, it may be
enlightening to consider more deeply this idea of spirit possession.
The Tibetans would suggest that we can become possessed by an
attachment to a past situation or emotion and that desire, hatred
and ignorance are at the root of all illness.

African writer Malidoma Some has shown that tribal practices
considered ignorant and superstitious may actually prove as effective as our much more sophisticated attempts at psychological
medicine. He shows how an attitude towards health which includes
a reverence to one's family, community and ancestors goes a long
way to create a healthy psychological environment. In illness, one

looks to the local herbalist but also to the village elders to address any problems in relationships which may be at the core of the imbalance. A village meeting may be held where disputes can be aired in a kind of group encounter session, facilitated by the shaman or village elder. He stresses ritual as vital in maintaining personal and community health, and considers that many of the problems facing Western culture stem from the abandonment of our rituals, which are an acceptable way to share our problems with others, and our loss of community:

> Alienation is one of the many faces of modernity. The cure is communication and community—a new sense of togetherness. By opening to each other, we diminish the pressure of being alone and exiled.[4]

Ageing and death

Malidoma Some suggests that our lack of respect and understanding of death has created a society which refuses to acknowledge the ageing process, preferring to prolong youth at all costs. As we fear death, and often refuse to talk about death, our death rituals are shallow and have no meaning. They do not serve the purpose for which they were intended—to create a safe passage to the next world for the deceased, and to give full vent to the grief of family and friends. Our inability to grieve may also impact on our health. According to the Chinese, who also have precisely formulated death rituals, unresolved grief affects the lungs and restricts the breath. The ability to breathe deeply reflects the ability to engage with life. Similarly the Yaqui tradition of Mexico suggests that without acknowledging death, one cannot fully live, that only by accepting the transience of life can one fully engage with the present moment.

The imbalances of our present day health care system may be partly due to our unbalanced view of life. In our well-meaning attempts to prolong life, we must be careful that we aim to prolong quality of life, not simply quantity. In our current medical system, the death of a patient is generally seen as a failure of the medical care teams to succeed in maintaining life. Current fears of the ulti-mate uncontrollable event in our lives lead us to expect the medical service to do everything in their power to prevent death. This situa-tion, which can result in a very poor quality of life for the sick patient, will deny the rights of the individual to be involved in their own process of treatment, or in the way they might choose to die. In order to understand health, we must examine our attitudes to our lives, and within this we must not avoid the discussion of death and the need to include the process of dying in that of life.

Intricately linked with our inability to accept death is our desper-ate attempt to ward off the ageing process. In our desire to prolong youth, psychologist James Hillman would suggest that we are deny-ing the role of elder and advisor that is so key to a balanced society:

> For centuries late years were associated not with dying but with vitality and character. The old were regarded as stable depositories of customs and legends, guardians of legal values, experts in skills and crafts, and valued voices in communal council. What mattered was force of char-acter proven by length of years.[5]

In our use of pharmaceutical drugs to delay menopause, we must be aware of the long-term effects both on our health and on society. According to Dr. Barbara Evans in her book *Life Change*:

> Some societies reward women for their services to the race when they reach the end of their fertility, giving them the freedom and often the status they had lacked during their reproductive years. Women from countries where age is venerated suffer less physically than other women at the change of life, or menopause. Unfortunately, ours is not one of those societies.[6]

That the pharmaceutical companies have played on the fears of women of becoming unattractive to men as they grow older is dis-cussed at length by Germaine Greer in *The Change*:

> In the guise of immense chivalrous sympathy for women destroyed by the tragedy of menopause, a group of male professionals, with the will-ing assistance of the pharmaceutical multinationals . . . (researched) the

possibility of eliminating menopause and keeping women both appetising and responsive to male demand from puberty to the grave, driving the dreaded old woman off the face of the earth for ever.[7]

Possibly most disturbing is her discussion of the first menopause clinics set up in South Africa by Dr. Wulf H. Utian after he 'happened' to be in West Berlin and was invited to visit a major multinational pharmaceutical firm. (Schering in Berlin produce 14 or 15 different kind of steroid drugs for women.) According to Dr. Utian:

> A new female hormone was mentioned and thereby started my interest in the subject. Upon my return to Cape Town . . . I spelled out my plans for a menopause clinic.[8]

The menopause was assigned 'disease status' in order to sell drugs. Of Dr. Wulf Utian's 26 papers published on menopause, further study showed them to be poorly designed and with an unacceptable degree of bias. Studies of his research in a menopause clinic in Glasgow showed no significant effect of the drugs above placebo, and no evidence of what Utian described as 'deficiency disease'. Before its wide-scale adoption by women, studies on Hormone Replacement Therapy were all funded by drug companies. Dr. Greer suggests:

> Traditionally women have not made a great fuss about menopause. . . . They medicated themselves when necessary with simple preparations of plant material according to the season. There is no agreement in this vast pharmacopoeia because it is entirely reliant upon microclimates. . . .[9]

Because all traditional systems agree that matter is imbued with spirit, it is the quality of the spirit which is seen as the most important single factor governing health and also the ageing process. Matter may naturally decline and decay, but it is spirit which keeps it alive and animated. Spirit provides the intelligence of our cells, it allows our cuts to heal and our bodies to repair. Attention to spirit therefore is of primary importance in traditional health and healing practices. Ayurvedic doctor Deepak Chopra suggests that we can slow down the ageing process, but with the help of meditation practices rather than pharmaceuticals.[10] The Chinese tradition has long searched for the 'pill of immortality', but the Chinese alchemical texts stress that it is in adopting meditation and exercise practices that this 'inner alchemy' is to be achieved.

The vital force and illness as a teacher

Within the Western tradition the concept of 'spirit' is considered to be crucial in all healing, and is often referred to as the life force or 'vital force'. Max Heindel (1865–1919) describes how this vital force radiates out of the 'vital body'. He suggests that if the spirit or vital force is strong, there is resistance to disease:

> In sickness, when the vital body is weak, these emanations do not readily eliminate disease germs. Therefore the danger of contracting disease is much greater when the vital forces are low than when one is in robust health.[11]

The philosophy behind natural medicine considers that it is this dynamic force that provides the energy to rebalance and restore the body to health. It is this vital force which directs all chemical and physical reactions within the body and maintains health. When energy is low, there is susceptibility to illness. In this model, illness may be seen as the most effective way for the body to alert the individual to an imbalance within the vital force. The reaction of the body to that imbalance will be the natural way for the body to heal itself. For example, under certain conditions inflammation may be the natural way for the body to create self-healing; swelling may be part of the mechanism used by the body to rid itself of a foreign microbe. The current conventional approach is to remove the symptom, for example the swelling, in order to bring relief. But to suppress the symptoms does not necessarily address the root of the illness. According to Robert Tisserand:

> If we recognize the existence of this life force, and that it is the only power which can produce health us, we will realize that we must work with it and not against it. We cannot heal directly; we can only help the body to help itself by encouraging the natural healing force within and allowing it to do

what it wants to do. So often we interpret sickness as something unfortunate and undesirable and yet often especially in acute disease, it is a manifestation of the body's attempt to restore health and harmony.[12]

In the *Organon of Medicine*, founder of homoeopathy Samuel Hahnemann suggests that the vital force present in the body actually creates the disagreeable sensations and abnormal functions that we call disease. He continues to explain that:

> the vital force can only reveal and express its untunement by pathological manifestations in feeling and function . . . i.e. the disease symptoms. [13]

The body is a unique indicator of what is happening to us within our environment. When we tip the balance too far, it results in ill-health. But we can learn from our illness, and it can be seen as an opportunity for growth and learning. Traditional systems of medicine aim to strengthen the body's own resistance and stimulate the body's own healing power to help regain a state of health. Ill health may therefore be seen as a sign that the body is working to repair itself. Good health is seen as our ability to return to a natural balance that we recognize to be our own. Optimum health is a state in which we have the ability to achieve balance with our external environment. Traditional systems of healing suggest that if we listen to our bodies, we can tune in to our internal environment and also develop awareness of our responses to the ecology of the exterior. Illness may still trigger fears from the past, where disease or injury did often lead to death. In a more contemporary context, illness will often evoke a sense of powerlessness and uncertainty. We feel uncomfortable sensations that we try to interpret. We will measure the body changes against our 'normal' state and in our attempt to explain what is going on we will compare ourselves to others with reference to similar social groupings, age, sex, etc. In an attempt to understand we will give names to the discomfort and create expectations for the recovery. However, if we see illness as a teacher, or as a response to changes that we have been unable to adapt to, then it should be possible to see a state of ill health as one that could be instructive and lead to a future state of improved health.

Native American healer Lea Bill (Rippling Water Woman) describes three stages of the healing process. The first involves prayers, the second focuses on healing the physical body 'using vibration and releasing negative imprinting and accumulated stress in the body', which in preference takes place in the open air. The third stage involves instruction and counselling to the client, to teach and provide guidance. Healing ceremonies of the Navaho are not just for healing the physical body, and illness is seen to be a unique time to tune in to spirit:

> Illness for the Navaho is the rare opportunity to intensify this journey to a deeper experience. It brings him to the source of his being, so that his brokenness can be transformed into intactness, so that our healing can encompass a reconciliation with our humanity beyond any question of just physical repair.[14]

By remaining aware of our connection to the earth, traditional systems of healing can help us to regain our connection to nature and the natural world. And by emphasizing that true health is a combination of body mind and spirit, traditional healing systems will help to heal the wounds of the spirit which deeply affect the health of society today. Complementary and Alternative Medicine, by keeping contact with the roots of health, can take us forward towards a state of health and wholeness.

Chapter 2

Health and Holism

Complementary and alternative medicine claims to treat the 'whole person', and is often referred to as 'holistic' health care. It has grown up in the shadow of a National Health Service which has become increasingly fragmented. As scientific knowledge grew throughout the past century, modern biomedicine became more specialized, and the body was divided into its various systems, each system having its specialists and hospital departments. Medical schools teach medicine in this way; the very scale and complexity of the knowledge available making it impossible to know all there is to know about the body. Specialization became the only way forward. Specialization and fragmentation was the inevitable outcome of a mechanistic approach to medicine, with the body divided into its component parts, and each of the individual parts of the 'machine' being manipulated chemically, removed surgically, or more recently a defective part being exchanged for a second-hand one.

> The science of medicine is still based on the notion of the body as a machine, of disease as the consequence of breakdown of the machine, and of the doctor's task as repair of the machine.[1]

Complementary and Alternative Medicine would suggest that it is the relationship between the parts that is missing, and that in its detailed study of the individual parts of the body, medicine was losing sight of the living dynamic whole. But it is this continual pursuit of smaller and smaller parts that has resulted the major breakthroughs of modern medicine. Throughout the last century we have seen the development of biochemistry, which rapidly established itself as the scientific basis of biomedicine. It is the understanding of the cell and its molecular mechanisms which has allowed the development of the drugs and vaccines on which much of biomedicine is based. Vaccines and antibiotics were developed in the early part of the 20th century; many of the psychoactive drugs, antidepressants and tranquillizers, were developed in the 1950s; while discoveries in endocrinology gave us an array of hormonal drugs including insulin, cortisone and the contraceptive pill. With the observed successes of many of these interventions, medical problems became reduced to a biochemical phenomena. The aim of the physician was reduced to finding the mechanism central to the problem, and once this mechanism was understood, to counteract it with a drug.

By acting in isolation in this way, there was a lack of attention to the actions of the substances on other parts of the system. Drug disasters such as 'Thalidomide' occurred when a drug to treat morning sickness during pregnancy was insufficiently tested to ensure that there would be no effect on the unborn child. The birth of thousands of deformed children went some way to ensure that the 'side effects' of drugs are clearly researched and labelled. It is the unwanted side effects of various molecular substances that give us some indication of the dangers of the fragmentation of modern medicine. Against this background of fragmentation, the words holism and holistic have been used to define the systems of health and healing which look at the whole of the body, not just the separate parts, and maintain that the whole is necessarily more than the sum of the parts.

Holism suggests that individual symptoms should not be seen in isolation, but rather may point to a pattern of disharmony throughout the system. A holistic approach to health suggests that the mind and the body are not separate, that mental and emotional imbalance will have a physical effect and vice versa. It suggests that an individual cannot be treated in isolation from his or her life circumstances, and that if health is to change, life habits and patterns may also have to change. It also suggests that mental attitude plays a decisive role in individual health. CAM looks for the cause of disease and maintains that unless the root of the problem is addressed cure will only be temporary. With its concentration on the molecular mechanisms of disease and their counteraction with drugs, conventional medicine has neglected the cause of disease and the whole area of preventive medicine.

Drawing both on ancient wisdom and modern innovation, CAM practitioners take into account the emotional, mental and spiritual nature of the patient, and encourage a view of the body as intelligent and self-healing. Some would suggest that alternative systems are concerned with the living body, while much of biomedicine is based on study of the dead. The dissection of cadavers which has given modern medicine its intricate knowledge of anatomy furthers this fragmentary approach by allowing in-depth study of the isolated part, while ignoring the 'life-force' or the 'patterns of information' which lie behind the physical form. Holistic health practitioners are concerned with the restoration and maintenance of health, and see the body as a whole with remarkable powers to restore, revitalize and to regenerate itself. These are the concerns and beliefs that should inform all medical practice.

Science and language

Complementary and alternative health practices may appeal to the individual patient because they adopt a language of wholeness and are able to look beyond symptoms to provide a framework to aid the understanding of the disease process. But these explanations generally appeal to the intuitive rather than the rational, to what may be called 'body knowing' rather than scientific fact. Within the clinical encounter, an individual may feel better, more confident, more at ease, without necessarily being able to analyse what has happened in a scientific or rational way. But in evaluating treatment, the medical and scientific community tends to dismiss subjective experience, putting its trust in objective scientific proof.

In order to create more efficient ways of evaluating our health and the effectiveness of various healing systems, maybe we need to question what it means to be objective and what is scientific proof.

Our culture places its trust in science to provide the truth, and yet the advances in modern physics throughout the last century created an environment in which the physicists were forced to question their view of reality and admit that objectivity was more difficult to achieve than had previously been imagined. Max Planck, often referred to as the father of quantum mechanics, said at the beginning of the last century:

> Science . . . means unresting endeavour and continually progressing development toward an aim which the poetic intuition may apprehend, but which the intellect can never fully grasp.[2]

In 1927 the most famous meeting of physicists in history took place in Copenhagen. This was part of an ongoing debate between Einstein and Neils Bohr in which Bohr maintained that it may never be possible to construct a single 'model of reality'.

> This acknowledgement is more than a recognition of the limitations of this theory or that theory. It is a recognition emerging throughout the West that knowledge itself is limited. Said another way, it is a recognition of the difference between knowledge and wisdom'.[3]

Inseparably related to the Copenhagen discussions is Neils Bohr's theory of complementarity. Much of modern physics grew out of Max Planck's attempts in the early 20th century to understand the nature of light. He discovered that light could be seen either as a wave or as a particle, and his findings formed the basis of inquiry for much of modern physics. Bohr suggested these inconsistencies occur because it is not light that we are measuring but our interaction with light. We can cause light to manifest its wave-like properties or its particle-like qualities depending on the particular experiment we choose to perform. Depending on our choice of methodology, we will get a given result. As Gary Zukov explains:

> Bohr's principle of complementarity also addresses the underlying relation of physics to consciousness. The experimenter's choice of experiment determines in which exclusive aspect the same phenomenon will manifest itself. Likewise Heisenberg's uncertainty principle demonstrates

that we cannot observe a phenomena without changing it. The physical properties which we observe in the 'external' world are enmeshed in our own perceptions not only psychologically, but ontologically as well.[4]

This suggests that not only do the experiments that we construct affect the outcome, but that our world view will affect the way that we interpret the results. We see what we expect to see. Although for many decades these discoveries remained within the realms of sub-atomic physics and seemed to have little relevance to the world of things and beings, the ideas of both complementarity and uncertainty have more recently made their mark. It is now understood, though not necessarily practised, that all scientific facts are inescapably predetermined by the theories and methods that generate their collection.

The science that informs most medical trials is based on an objective quantitative approach. It values objective, quantitative procedures above subjective and qualitative ones. According to James Oschman this is so fundamental to those involved in medical science that it is 'like the air we breathe, virtually invisible to those of us who conduct scientific enquiry', though he proceeds to add that one aspect of science is to continually review and challenge current scientific method.

> What science holds to be the truth has radically changed throughout the ages. Science continually reviews itself and the 'scientific method'. Currently objective, quantitative procedures are considered superior to subjective and qualitative procedures.[5]

Oschman also points out that the subject chosen for research, and the way in which the research project is structured, will be based on the philosophical assumptions of the scientist, and that theories and methods create the facts. J. W. Radcliffe, philosopher of science at Berkeley, suggests:

> . . . that there is no basis for our widely held belief that qualitative and quantitative approaches are opposites, dichotomous, mutually exclusive, or even separable. From all perspectives, all approaches to enquiry are inherently qualitative, subjective in nature.[6]

He goes on to explain that within any experiment the scientist must first decide to follow a specific line of enquiry, and to define the problem in a particular way; to select the instruments that will be used, and to decide which method of data collection to employ etc. The interpretation of the data will also be determined by the context in which the results are examined. Radcliffe continues:

> For example, a whole line of research may be started because of the current status of research support—which areas are being funded. . . . A hidden goal may be to produce results of a sort that will be well received and therefore given to further funding, or that will bring attention to the investigator and to his or her favourite theory.[7]

That much of complementary and alternative medicine lacks scientific verification we can begin to attribute to the limitations of current scientific medical enquiry rather than the failings of the medicine itself. The very nature of CAM is its concern with the whole. Currently, medical science only has ways to measure the parts. By exposing CAM to these conventional research methodologies we run the risk of losing the very essence of holistic health care. This can already be seen in the trials carried out on both acupuncture and herbal medicine. An early acupuncture trial used stimulation to the acupuncture point *nei guan* to test its effectiveness in post operative nausea. Although nausea and vomiting are one indication for the use of this point, there are many others, including heart pain, chest pain, and because of its direct connection with the heart, a trained acupuncturist would use it with caution, and nearly always in combination with other points to create an individual treatment. The project was described as 'inconclusive'. In a later project a research team at Oxford Medical centre in the late 1980s invited a Chinese medical doctor to conduct research, using traditional methods of diagnosis and treatment. The results were markedly different, showing considerable improvement, and the project was given serious attention by the medical profession.[8] And while the herbalist will maintain that the efficacy of a herb is dependent on using the herb in its entirety, and often in its combination with other herbs (that the effect of the whole is definitely greater than the sum of its parts) the drug companies are busy isolating an individual active ingredient and researching its effect on particular aspects of our chemical metabolism. There is not much money to be made from research into the action of the whole herb, or a formula made of a combination of many herbs, because plants are not patentable.

While the various therapies undergo double blind trials and various other possibly already outdated modes of enquiry, maybe we should move our attention to the development of new research methodologies. The so called 'soft sciences' already employ qualitative types of research, but within medicine, objective quantitative study is given precedence. Medicine needs to include the methods of soft science to measure the effectiveness of the various therapies and medicines in ways that will include quality of life and subjective experience. Meanwhile, how we can begin to look at the mechanisms of therapies such as acupuncture and homoeopathy which claim to work with the body's subtle energy systems? And how can we begin to understand the role of consciousness on health? These are the questions that science needs to be asking. MD Richard Gerber suggests:

> The current model of medicine is still Newtonian in character, for pharmokinetic therapy is based upon a biomolecular/mechanistic approach. . . . The healing arts must be updated with new insights from the world of physics and other allied sciences.[9]

It has been within the biosciences rather than physics that a new approach to science has emerged. Systems theory, developed originally to study 'a set of elements standing in relation', may allow us to study the body as a whole and the individual in relationship to the environment.

The pattern that connects

According to Gregory Bateson, science never proves anything, it only probes. He maintains that our civilization is based deep in the illusion of objective reality, and that all knowledge is essentially subjective. It was Fritjof Capra's meeting with Gregory Bateson at a conference in Boulder, Colorado in 1976 (when Bateson famously exclaimed 'Capra? The man is crazy! He thinks we are all electrons!'[10]) that led Capra to embrace systems theory as the most appropriate tool to study the paradigm shift taking place in all the sciences. As a particle physicist, Fritjof Capra had become fascinated with the apparent connection between the world view postulated by sub-atomic physics and the various philosophical systems of the East. He particularly cited Taoism, and in 1977 published *The Tao of Physics*, which became the first of many books to explore this relationship. He felt that the discoveries of modern physics would expand into other sciences, creating a new model of reality and a framework to explain much of the 'unexplainable'. Gregory Bateson disagreed. Bateson's interest was in what he called 'the pattern that connects'. He described physics as cold and inanimate; as a biologist, his interest was in understanding living systems. Bateson pointed out that there was a fundamental difference between living and non-living things; his exploration was of the world of 'living process', where order arises from patterns of information flow rather than from physical relationships of cause and effect, and where differences in quality are more profoundly important than differences in quantity.[11] The language of systems theory fits well with the experience of healing and holism. As physics is playing its part in questioning the old mechanistic paradigm, systems theory may provide a key to the science and language for the new.

According to Bertalanffy, who originally proposed systems theory:

> It seems to be the most serious shortcoming of classical occidental philosophy, from Plato to Descartes and Kant, to consider man primarily as a spectator, as *ens cogitans*, while for biological reasons, he has essentially to be a performer, as *ens agens*, in the world he is thrown in.[12]

Systems theory seeks to understand relationships and situations; it aims to provide a more general and approximate understanding of the world. It is concerned with the study of organisms or living things, with processes of organization and integration. A living system is defined by its ability for 'self-organization' and also 'self-replication'. So a cell is a living system, as are various tissues of the human body. A living system retains its identity by changing to adapt to its environment. It is able to remain stable by constant change and modification. According to Brian Goodwin, "living systems create and are created by their environment even on a cellular level."[13] Within the cell there is a perpetual exchange of information/nutrients/waste matter between the cell and the extracellular matrix. Each cell of the body is an independent 'whole', capable of self-organization and also of self-replication, but it is also a part of a greater whole, for example a liver, which is also part of a greater whole, and so on. Arthur Koestler coined the term 'holon' to describe the individual parts of the system, which themselves make up a greater whole. According to Koestler, each holon has a basic polarity—looking inward it sees itself as a self-contained unique whole; looking outward it sees itself as a dependent part. He suggests that there is a dynamic equilibrium between these two forces which creates life.

Homoeostasis and adaptation

Homoeostasis is the term used to describe the state of dynamic equilibrium within a living system. It describes a condition which may vary but which is relatively constant. The human body, for example, is constantly changing and adapting to remain relatively constant. This is self-regulation, which is carried out by a complex series of both negative and positive feedback loops. In this way the structure and function of the body are maintained. Adaptation implies the ability to change according to external circumstances and also an ability for creative evolution.

For example, within a very safe protected environment an organism may flourish for a certain time, but will lack external stimuli for change, adaptation and growth. On the other hand a changing complex environment will present challenges which must be met by flexible behaviour. But if the challenge exceeds a critical limit there may be a major crisis, which could lead to degeneration, stagnation, or sudden extinction. Depending on the ability of the organism to adapt, this threat to survival could possibly lead to major reorganization within the system, allowing the system to function more efficiently. Illness can been viewed in a similar way—certain symptoms being seen as the attempt of the organism to adapt to a new environment or situation. If the system is unable to adapt, there may be a more serious breakdown of function. It is a situation of breakdown or breakthrough. And again the language of systems theory echoes that of healing.

The definition of holism in the *Concise Oxford Dictionary* is as follows: "The tendency in nature to form wholes that are more than the sum of the parts by creative evolution." This definition provides an interesting juxtaposition of the words creative and evolution. It suggests a progressive movement or unfoldment that could be both 'creationist' and evolutionary. It suggests that the world came into being, and continues to come into being by both adaptation and moments of sudden creative change. This concept of order out of apparent chaos is central to systems thinking. Coherent systems are said to 'emerge' from the interactions between their component elements, and apparently chaotic behaviour at one level can give rise to order at another. Brian Goodwin suggests:

> Whereas physicists have dealt with 'simple' systems . . . biologists deal with systems (cells, organisms) that are hideously complex, with thousands of different types of gene and molecule all interacting in different ways. . . . A particularly striking property of these complex systems is that even chaotic behaviour at one level of activity, molecules or cells or organisms, can give rise to distinctive order at the next level, morphology and behaviour. This has resulted in one of the primary recurring themes of complex studies: order emerges out of chaos.[14]

Alternative practitioners have long maintained that physical illness may be a sign to the organism of the need for change; many of those who work with patients in crisis discuss the potential for breakthrough. Professor William Tiller of Stamford University has suggested that illness can be part of a "biofeedback mechanism for the transformation of man." [15] In this article he suggests that illness is used by the organism to facilitate this leap to a higher level of organization. This is obviously part of the evolutionary process, but also an important aspect of health and healing.

The language of systems theory consistently mirrors the language of holistic health. As this language seeps into the consciousness, and more scientific credence is given to the study of the whole as well as the parts, holistic healing will find its voice. According to Julian Silverman:

> Our current use of language promotes a view that the world is made up of separate things. We are taught to memorize the names of the parts, rather than to think of how they fit together. This does not facilitate the perception of the relativistic, interrelated, integrated nature of reality. [16]

Systems theory begins to give a language to those concepts which are familiar to the alternative health field such as wholeness, integration, cooperation, balance, harmony, sufficiency, integrity, sharing. It gives credence to the fundamental message of holism— that disease in any part of the body has but one function—to alert the whole to an imbalance within itself. Systems theory helps us to give value to the relationship between the parts, to the pattern that connects, and also the importance of dynamic change and transformation.

Body-mind

During the later part of the 20th century, both physicists and biologists were suggesting that it is in the study of consciousness that the next breakthrough in science will occur. This is no easy task, as the old criteria of objective and quantitative science cannot be used to study consciousness. Psychiatrist R. D. Laing suggested that the challenge of this current century is the synthesis of what we observe and quantify from without and what we know and qualify from within. [17]

Mind/body separation is at the heart of the dualism upheld by conventional medicine, and it creates the most serious block to understanding health. Even though most GPs would admit that stress can play an important part in various pathologies, the study and understanding of mental and physical health remains quite separate. Even within CAM, although there is an acceptance and in many cases a complete philosophy based on mind/body interconnection, we have a long way to go before we understand the true nature of consciousness.

In a recent article entitled 'The Psychologizing of Chinese Healing Practices in the United States',[18] Linda Barnes suggests that during the 30 years or so in which Chinese medicine has flourished within the USA, Western practitioners have stressed the importance of emotional and mental factors in diagnosis and treatment of disease. Her study focused on 200 practitioners within the Boston area, and she suggests an emphasis in treatment on the relationship between illness states and the emotional life of the individual. Many practitioners are blending psychotherapeutic skills with acupuncture or herbal treatment, others suggest that acupuncture treatment can eliminate the need for psychotherapy altogether. Many of these practitioners refer to mental, emotional or spiritual causative factors of illness, which are in turn connected to 'energy blockages'. Such terminology also informs popular psychological models which describe the individual as 'stuck', blocked, or in need of 'letting go'.

One of the most interesting aspects of her research was the differences recorded while talking to Chinese practitioners, who did not tend to discuss mental and emotional factors. She mentions that during a conference in which a party of delegates from Beijing medical college presented their research, they were asked about the treatment of psychological problems. She describes how the doctors went into a huddle from which they finally emerged to answer that they did not understand the question. Dr. Steven Birch suggested that they did not understand the question because to them illness was seen as an imbalance of *qi*. Whether that imbalance manifested physically or mentally was immaterial to their diagnosis and treatment.

Mental health and physical health are organized by two separate authorities within the USA, and research is funded by either the National Institute for Health or the National Institute for Mental Health. Candace Pert, a Research Professor within the department of Physiology and Biophysics at Georgetown University Medical Centre in Washington DC, discovered the drug Peptide T, which claims to block the access of the HIV virus to the receptor cells. Her team ran into problems for many reasons. Firstly their research was into chemicals usually associated with the brain and therefore considered to be within the realm of mental health. This created problems of credibility for the research itself, and also with funding. Candace Pert suggests:

> . . . underlying all of it was a fundamental but less visible drama—the shift from old paradigm to new paradigm. Conceived by believers in the mind-body connection, Peptide T was truly a child of the new, more holistic paradigm. And that was a big problem for a large establishment institution.[19]

What follows was possibly more sinister. In her book *Molecules of Emotion*, Dr. Pert writes about the discovery of Peptide T and her attempts to get the drug accepted by the medical establishment. At that time huge sums of money were available for AIDS research, and there was a race to get a drug on the market. The drug AZT was also being developed within the same institution, and it competed for funding. AZT had been developed as a cancer drug with a chemotherapeutic effect, which means that it destroys the body's healthy cells as well as the cells of the virus. Despite its obvious side effects and its short-term effectiveness, due to tolerance, the government decided to fund AZT. At the same time a Boston-based research team, funded by a private bio-tech company, announced that Peptide T was ineffective as his team had been unable to replicate the results. Dr. Pert admits:

> I was completely unprepared to deal with the kind of real-world, big-business wheeling and dealing that was necessary if I was going to have any hope of having a direct impact on people's health.

Candace Pert's early research into neuropeptides determined that mood-altering chemicals formerly thought to have been exclusive to brain activity could be found in various other cells of the body. The chemicals themselves are proving to be of great interest in providing vital links between the mind and the body, the emotions and our states of health. This work, usually known as 'psychoneuro-endocrinology' has been utilized by Deepak Chopra to provide scientific background to his theories of mind-body connection. A medical doctor and Ayurvedic practitioner, Chopra claims that true healing takes place at the 'quantum' level, and that these most subtle levels of nature hold the greatest potential energy. It is here Chopra suggests that thoughts and emotions have their effect on the physical body:

> A neuropeptide springs into existence with the touch of a thought . . . [20]

He proposes a 'quantum mechanical body' which is the underlying basis for everything that we are: thoughts, emotions, proteins, cells, organs . . . According to Chopra our whole body is intelligent, our whole body thinks and our whole body feels. (Our skin can be sad; our livers depressed.) It is not just a brain phenomenon. In his view all healing takes place through consciousness. Our body-consciousness knows how to heal a cut, mend a broken bone. In his view it just takes a bit more work to reverse cancers, or even slow down the ageing process.

The work of Dr. Carl Simonton with cancer patients is just one example of the way in which a change in consciousness or awareness can help the body to heal. Simonton suggests that changing people's belief systems about cancer is the most important step in reversing their illness. He uses relaxation techniques and guided imagery through which patients are made to feel more in control of their disease, less powerless. Cancer is shown to be less as an external powerful agent, more as a rather stupid, bumbling overgrowing part of themselves. Simonton suggests that the belief system of patient and physician crucial for healing. His work aims to activate motivation to get well, and he suggests that the patient must believe that he or she can get well. His methods are complementary, in that they may utilize positive meditation on radiotherapy treatment.[21]

In his preface to Candace Pert's *Molecules of Emotion*, Deepak Chopra suggests:

> Her pioneering research has demonstrated how our internal chemicals and their receptors are the actual biological underpinnings of our awareness and consciousness, validating what Eastern philosophers, shamans, rishis and alternative practitioners have known and practised for centuries. The body is not a mindless machine; the body and mind are one.

Chapter Three

The Web of Healing

In its tendency to specialize and fragment, our health care system has failed to provide answers to the increasing variety of health problems which involve the whole body rather than its parts. Illnesses such as chronic fatigue syndrome and irritable bowel syndrome are not consistent with any measurable pathology, and were dismissed as being 'all in the mind' for many years. (The vagueness of the names suggest how poorly they are understood.) Michael Hyland, Professor of Health Psychology at the University of Plymouth, proposes that conventional medicine is unable to address these types of pathology as it is not 'specific pathology'. He suggests that there is also a kind of 'network pathology' which can produce a variety of symptoms which are often difficult to define or measure, and it is therefore difficult for them to be treated by conventional methods. Specific pathologies tend to generate particular signs and symptoms which can be measured by conventional diagnostic methods. He goes on to suggest that it is because Complementary and Alternative Medicine sees the body as a whole, that it is able to treat network pathology.

> Complexity theory now shows us that the properties of some complex systems—networks in particular—cannot be attributed to individual components but emerge from whole systems. So why shouldn't disease emerge from the body in a similar way? If so, conventional medicine will never be enough to cure all our ills. And the assumptions of CAM may not be as unscientific as they seem.[1]

Professor Hyland goes on to suggest that the body, as a complex system, is self-regulating, and inherent within any self-regulating system is the ability to learn to self-regulate more effectively. Complementary and alternative therapies work with this self-regulating system, enabling the system to re-learn what it has forgotten, and possibly guiding towards more effective self-regulation. Within many disciplines of CAM there is an aspect of 'teaching' the body— whether by structural realignment as with Alexander Technique, or with subtle treatments such as homoeopathy and acupuncture which teach the body by directly addressing the information system. If the body can learn, then the body can learn more efficient self-regulation. Conventional medicine takes away the power of the organism to self-regulate, and therefore diminishes its ability to learn and could be considered to be against evolution. For example, anti-inflammatory drugs given for asthma may help the symptoms for a short time, but if the drugs are withdrawn the inflammation returns, often more severely. Similarly, steroid creams used for eczema may bring an apparently miraculous decrease in symptoms, but withdrawal of the cream will exacerbate them. In both cases there is no 'cure', only a suppression of symptoms which reappear as soon as the suppressing agent is taken away. CAM would suggest that in the suppression of symptoms the underlying imbalance will manifest itself at a deeper level of the organism.

Each individual therapy within the CAM umbrella will have its own philosophy of health, its own view of symptoms, networks and self-regulation. There is much diversity, but also they also have much in common. The differences may be seen as a reflection of each specific area of expertise. Working directly with the physical body, an osteopath will see the body primarily in terms of its structure, while an acupuncturist working with the *qi* will be attempting to tune in to the subtle energy. A homoeopath will become particularly skilled at recognizing types of character and relating that to disease patterns; a herbalist will develop an affinity with the plants he or she uses in daily practice, so that they become like friends and familiars, resonating with various systemic imbalances. Each viewpoint has its own merit, each has a part of the truth. Each individual therapist will develop very different skills which enable them to diagnose and treat a variety of ailments. The extent to which any thera-peutic encounter is 'holistic' must depend on several factors, not merely the type of therapy practised. It is not so much a matter of which therapies are more holistic, but how they are used. The out-come may be dependent on both the therapist's ability to under-stand a problem on many levels and the patient's ability to respond.

As we look in more detail at the most commonly used therapies within the growing field of CAM, let us think of what each has to offer; to offer in the realm of treatment of symptoms, to offer the body in expanding its self-regulating ability and also to widen our view of health and healing. We will not discuss each discipline in depth, but attempt to give some kind of framework for their inter-relationships. And rather than attempting to create a single 'model of reality' of the healing process, we need to employ some 'boot-strap thinking', allowing each discipline to take its place and hold its own wisdom. We will introduce each therapy according to its mode of intervention within the bodymind continuum, while bearing in mind not only that this is a simplification but also that in the holis-tic world view, stimulation to any part must effect the whole.

Structure = function

Both osteopathy and chiropractic suggest that by manipulating the structure of the body there will be an effect on the function. Treatment aims to restore the symmetry of the body that has been lost by life's various trauma. For example an accident or an opera-tion will tend to push the body out of alignment, and we then hold these patterns of tension in our structure. Many practitioners would also suggest that emotional shocks are held in the body in the same way, and that working with the physical structure can also help to release the emotional trauma.

The Western tradition has recorded many forms of manipulation: the Greek healer Asclepiades wrote about rubbing the spine to cure all ills, and both traction and walking on the back are recorded in Greek medical texts. Later in Europe, the church declared these manipulative techniques to be 'bizarre, superstitious and immoral'. During the middle ages, clicking the back or neck was the favoured way to expel demons, and in 1563 the 'manipulation of vertebrae' was denounced as the work of the devil. With the rise of surgery, many of these techniques fell into disrepute, but practices such as bone setting and back walking remained in a hidden form throughout Europe. Lumbago was said to be cured by a woman, preferably a virgin or a mother of twins, walking on the back. And we can see that vestiges of both these techniques and the superstitious attitudes towards them remain to the present day.

Osteopathy and chiropractic both use the structure of the body as a staring point towards a general theory of illness and disease. Both were founded in America in the later part of the 19th century, though they obviously draw on more ancient forms of healing. Opposed to the brutal techniques of the medicine of his time, Andrew Taylor Still (1828–1917) became interested in 'magnetic healing' and later 'bonesetting'. His experience with both techniques led him to believe that correct spinal alignment was vital to health, and a breakthrough came when treating a woman with asthma he noticed a misalignment of the upper spine. Manipulation of the upper vertebrae and ribs cured the asthma. Still went on to develop the practice of osteopathy, which aims to treat structure to affect function. He suggested that misplaced spinal bones are often the cause of functional problems and stressed the importance of keeping open channels of blood, lymph and cerebrospinal fluids, allowing body tissues to breathe or absorb nutrients as well as to eliminate waste products.

Chiropractic (literally hand practice, or manipulation) was developed in the US just a few years after osteopathy. Now the second largest primary health care treatment after orthodoxy, it is especially recognized in the USA, where it has largely supplanted osteopathy. Its concerns are the musculo-skeletal system and its relationship to the nervous system. It is similar to osteopathy, although there are some differences in manipulative techniques. Its founder Daniel David Palmer was a non-medical anatomist. He is said to have cured a case of sudden deafness by adjusting an upper dorsal vertebra. Palmer assumed that there had been some kind of nerve interference in the spine and went on to develop chiropractic, which proposes an intimate connection between the structure of the body and the nervous function.

Both techniques were dismissed by orthopaedic surgeons at the time, and are still dismissed by the majority today, even though modern medicine can offer little but rest and painkilling or anti-inflammatory drugs for a back problem, and both osteopathy and chiropractic have given relief to many where no other help has been offered. Both professions demand a rigorous training, and within the UK both are fully registered and teaching courses are fully accredited. In the words of Still:

> Remember you have been treated and dismissed as incurable by all kinds of doctors before coming to us, and if we help you at all we do more than others have done.[2]

William Garner Sutherland took the principles of osteopathy further when he recognized the potential for movement between the bones of the adult skull, and discovered a deep regular pulse throughout the body which is related to the subtle movement of cerebrospinal fluids. According to osteopath Sibyl Grundberg:

> It is this slow fluid rhythm, which Sutherland called the Involuntary Mechanism, that forms the basis of Osteopathic work in the cranial field, an osteopathic approach which takes into account the influence of cranial dynamics and fluid dynamics upon all the tissues of the body.[3]

Sutherland suggested that by regulating this involuntary mechanism in areas where it has been disturbed it may be possible to release tensions by harnessing the body's own self-balancing and self-healing powers. An extremely gentle and non-invasive technique, cranial osteopathy is often used on very small babies, particularly where there may have been birth trauma.

A practitioner of osteopathy or chiropractic will not only realign the bodily structure but bring the imbalance into conscious awareness, and teach ways to maintain alignment by awareness, exercise and posture. Similarly, Alexander Technique seeks to teach the individual to release tension and create a healthy structural balance. Alexander practitioners are 'teachers': their aim is to bring their clients to an awareness of their bodily imbalances and to help them to correct old postural habits. Frederick Matthias Alexander embarked on a process of self-healing which demanded developing awareness and changing life-long bodily habits. He realized that a pattern of misalignment ran throughout his whole body, and assumed that once he had found the root cause of his problem that it would be easy enough to rectify. But the habits of the body are difficult to break.

The aim of Alexander Technique is primarily to bring awareness. It aims to keep the individual free from any unnecessary tension. And while it may be easy enough to do this within the structure of the lesson, it is maintaining this in daily life which is both its challenge and its strength. Alexander Technique assumes that we have a sixth sense, a kinaesthetic sense which informs us of our position in space. Alexander teachers aim to increase conscious awareness of this sense. Body awareness, once developed, will enable us to correct minor imbalances before they become habits, we may learn to relax our shoulders, release our jaws before we develop a headache. Teaching here does not need to be verbal. The body recognizes healthy patterns of behaviour and various manipulative therapies nudge the body into self-awareness.

Massage is one of the earliest recorded forms of healing, and although it went out of favour in Europe during the Christian era, it has enjoyed a continuous history in the East. It has been recorded as far back as 500 BC in China, though no doubt dates from much earlier. Throughout Asia, massage is part of everyday life. In Japan, a visit to a bath house, still the most common way of bathing until very recently, would usually include exchanging shoulder massage with your neighbour. There is an interesting anecdote in the diaries of Captain Cook. Whilst in Tahiti he experienced 'a sort of rheumatic pain in one side from my hip to my foot' which had been troubling him for at least six months. He describes how a group of native women squeezed and pounded him for an hour, upon which he gained immediate relief. After three sessions he was completely cured. Massage has slowly begun to regain some status in the West, though Europe still lags way behind the USA in acceptance of its therapeutic effects. In the USA 11% of the population used therapeutic massage in 1998, compared to just over 1% in the UK in 1999.[4] Massage is defined as the use of any kind of pressure, kneading or rubbing of the body. Japanese *shiatsu* massage utilizes the acupuncture meridian system and is actually performed through light clothing. Massage therapy can fall into different categories of action, depending on the particular focus of the practitioner and the expectations of the client. Though ranging from sports massage to help recovery from injury, to intuitive massage to work on emotional blocks, the most common use of massage today is for the release of stress and tension. A more recent development is the use of massage and bodywork in relationship with psychotherapy. Here, specific trauma are dealt with by working on the body with stress release and with psychotherapeutic techniques.

Naturopathy

According to Naturopathy, health is dependent on being in harmony with nature, and it suggests the use of the elements of nature such as air, light, water, food and rest to regain health. Naturopathy maintains that only nature heals, and that it will heal if it is given the opportunity. It sees the body as self-healing, self-cleansing and self-regulating, suggesting that we are predisposed to good health, and that colds and flus are merely messengers from our body to let us know that we are out of balance. It is up to us to address that imbalance. In our natural state, we know what is good for us. We know instinctively which foods will be of benefit and which will not, but our habits, often built up over a lifetime, interfere with these natural abilities. A naturopath will look at the state of our hair, our eyes, our skin and our nails to see how well we are nourished. They will often assess body type and the state of balance of the four humours according to the tradition of Galenical medicine. Our needs will differ according to our body type: some may need more protein in the diet, others more carbohydrate. No one diet is good for all. Always stressed is the need to adapt lifestyle, to be willing to change patterns of work and rest, diet and exercise. Fasting is one of the techniques used in naturopathy as part of the need for rest. Our digestive systems are often overloaded and it is by resting and giving more time for the elimination of toxins that we can create a more efficient digestive system. We tend to resort easily to vitamins and supplements when possibly an overloaded system does not allow us to absorb. It is suggested that our modern diet is so lacking in nutrition that we need to supplement it with vitamins and minerals. But naturopathy would suggest that we should do all that we can to ensure that our food supply is improved, before resorting to supplements.

Often used as foundation for other therapies, naturopathy aims to restore balance, to work with nature and to aid the natural self-healing abilities of the body. A naturopath will often prescribe a regime to include diet and exercise, or possibly fasting and rest. Each individual will require a different system of healing, and that will change as the circumstances change. A naturopath may also recommend herbal treatment, or refer on to a herbalist.

Herbalism

Herbalism is the oldest form of medicine known to humankind. Ancient Egyptian writings refer to the medicinal use of 85 herbs, and the Greek writings of Dioscorides list over 400. The Greek's understanding of herbal medicine was lost to medieval Europe, but this wealth of knowledge was preserved within the Arab world, and re-introduced by the Moors into Southern Spain in the 10th century. Within continental Europe the old Greek or Galenic approach to herbalism has flourished since that time. In Britain, however, herbalism fell into disrepute, partly due to its association with superstitions and witchcraft, and it was not until the late 19th century that it reemerged with a strong influence from northern America. Nowadays, herbs may be used from the European, Indian or Ayurvedic, Chinese and North and South American traditions. Whatever tradition we study, our knowledge of plants has been handed down by our ancestors. In many cultures, plant medicine is the domain of the shaman. From the language of the Siberian Evenki, the word shaman means one who is both a singer and a seer. The shaman is able to 'see' the plant and understand its healing properties. The 'shaman-healer' will contact the spirit of the plant, and only then will be able to understand its properties and use the plant effectively.

According to Cherokee legend, it was the animals who brought disease to humankind, to halt their spread over the earth. But the plant kingdom found out and summoned a council at which they decided to provide people with all they needed to overcome this affliction brought to them by the animals.

People have always used plants for healing, and the modern biomedical pharmacopeia contains many drugs isolated from plant sources. Scientific medicine is able to work with these single identifiable chemicals as they are stable and can be tested in the laboratory, but herbalists maintain that it is by using the whole plant that real healing can take place. According to herbalist Andrew Chevallier:

> The whole herb is worth more than the sum of its parts and scientific research is increasingly showing that the active constituents of many herbs, for example, those in gingko (*Gingko biloba*) interact in complex ways to produce the therapeutic effect of the remedy as a whole. Plants contain hundreds if not thousands of different constituent chemicals that interact in complex ways. Frequently, we simply do not know in detail how a particular herb works—even though its medicinal benefit is established.[5]

Science is not yet sufficiently sophisticated to understand the synergistic effects of the many chemical compounds that make up a plant. And although the effects of single plants may be part of the folklore of most countries, it is the true art of the herbalist to understand how plants work together—in understanding not only the complex actions of a single plant, but also the effect of different plants used together in prescription. Andrew Chevallier suggests that the human body is much better suited to treatment with herbal remedies than with isolated chemical medicines. We have co-evolved with plants, and plants have formed the major part of our diet for thousands of years. Our digestive systems are used to plant material, and in many cases there is very little distinction between food and medicine. Many of our common foods—for example lemons, onions, oats and garlic—have medicinal properties. The distinction between food and medicine is very fine, and many herbs used in cooking, such as thyme, rosemary and sage, were originally used for their medicinal properties.

Herbal medicine works in a systemic way. Herbs are classified according to their function on a particular system of the body. Though often quite 'specific' in their actions, a prescription of herbal medicines aims to help the body's own healing abilities, rather than suppress symptoms. If there is a fever, a remedy such as elderflower (*Sambucus nigra*) may be prescribed to promote sweating, the body's natural way to deal with a fever. The aim of all herbal formulae is to create a balance between the individual ingredients, with the 'side effects' or toxicity of any specific single herb being regulated within the formula. The herbalist creates a formula to suit an individual rather than to treat a condition. The aim is not to suppress symptoms, but to strengthen the body system, which then enhances the body's ability to heal itself.

Essential oils

Essential oils are volatile oils distilled from plant material. They are found in seeds, roots, leaves and flowers. Stills for collecting essential oils found in the Indus Valley have been dated around 3000 BC, and there is evidence of their use in Sumeria and Egypt. As far back as the Egyptian civilization, four specific areas of usage have been documented. Olibanum (frankincense), myrrh, cedar and cypress were burnt to create an atmosphere of contemplation, to clear the head and to elevate the spirit. Oils such as cardamom, fennel, dill and coriander have been used as digestives to eliminate intestinal gas, whereas spice oils such as black pepper, star anis, cinnamon and clove stimulate the production of digestive enzymes, reduce poisoning and promote intestinal flora. Many spice oils are bactericidal. Oils such as eucalyptus, pine and niaouli have been used for the treatment of respiratory problems by inhalation or rubbing into the skin. The fourth category of oils is those used for perfumes, oils such as ylang ylang, jasmine, sandalwood, vetyver can be blended with a carrier oil and applied to the skin or added to the bath. These will complement the body's natural odours. Each oil will have its effect on the mind and emotions, and oils may be specifically blended for use in mental and emotional problems. Rose is an example of an oil which can cross boundaries and works on all four of the above levels. Rose essential oil has been treasured throughout history, its worth often valued above gold. 1000 roses are required to produce 1 gram of essential oil.

Modern aromatherapy is a blend of all these various aims and functions. Training in the UK tends to stress the use of essential oils as an adjunct to massage, and the calming relaxing qualities of the oils. The recent proliferation of training programmes emphasize the massage qualification, with a basic training in the use of the oils. The official registering bodies are now amalgamating to ensure a higher standard of training. By way of contrast, in France essential oils have been the subject of scientific research, and are considered to be so potent that they can only be prescribed by doctors and pharmacists. The oils are usually taken internally. Dr Paul Balaiche, chair of phytotherapy at the University of Paris Nord, has conducted a series of double blind trials with essential oils in the treatment of cystitis.[6] During a typical consultation he will take a urine sample and test up to seventy different essential oils on cultures of the urine. He will observe which oils have the effect of killing specific bacteria and create a blend of oils which may be made into pessaries, suppositories or mixed with ground herbs to make capsules. Essential oils such as niaouli *(Melaleuca viridiflora)* have been used in hospitals in France and Switzerland for their antibacterial effects. Dr. Balaiche will use the oils in much the same way as conventional drugs, but he would argue that as essential oils are extremely complex compounds, if they are applied correctly they will not cause side-effects and bacteria will not develop tolerance to them.

French naturopath and aromatherapist Patric Collin suggests that each method has its uses and is also open to abuse.[7] The use and effect of essential oils depend on the method and intention of the practitioner. For example, a common essential oil such as thyme (thymol) may be used symptomatically in order to get rid of bacteria. It may also be used naturopathically to stimulate the immune system and calm the parasympathetic nervous system, warming if there is cold. Psychologically the oil will give stability, strengthening without being too stimulating, and is recommended for those with an introverted nature. When choosing essential oils it is therefore important that the oil should be chosen with all these properties in mind. Tea tree oil, for example, will have an antiviral effect and will also stimulate the immune system. But it will be particularly well indicated if a problem is slow to heal and lingering, and the individual is feeling emotionally held back by circumstances.

Essential oils are created within the plant by the action of the sun. Any attempt to harvest oil when there has been no sunshine during the past 24 hours will show that no oils are produced. Essential oils may be considered to store the energy of the sun, and imprint it with the properties of the plant. They are the essence of the plant, and depending on the nature of the plant may be harmless or quite irritant to the skin. Care should always be taken, and oils are generally used in dilution.

Flower remedies

Flower remedies contain the 'energetic imprint' of the flower. Flowering parts are picked at the height of their maturity, and laid on a crystal bowl of spring water. They are left in the sunshine for 2-3 hours until the energy of the plant is captured by the water. According to Julian Barnard of Healing Herbs, spring water is used because it is completely fresh, the point of emergence from the earth being the equivalent of birth. 'When something is reborn it takes on the imprint of that which it touches'. The water is therefore able to take on the energetic imprint of the flowers.

Dr. Edward Bach was possibly one of the first to propose the psychologically healing power of illness. A medical doctor, Bach spent many years investigating the role of bacteriology in chronic disease. After working on the development of vaccines he became interested in homoeopathic principles. Through his many years of research he became aware that though exposed to the same bacteria and the same medical treatment, some people get better while others die. His observations led him to the belief that our emotional imbalances are the real cause of disease and that there are basic personality types which are related to patterns of ill health. He looked to nature to help heal these emotional imbalances, and in 1930 finally renounced his medical career to put his energy into this research. He left London and began his search for the plants that he believed held the answer to healing our emotional problems. He identified twelve deep states of emotional imbalance, which he described as twelve 'soul types', and in twelve years he found the twelve flowers that he felt reflected both the negative and positive aspect of these states, the life lesson of each soul type.

To classify the twelve types, Bach drew on both the Greek system of the four humours, with the four basic personality types of phlegmatic, choleric, melancholic and sanguine. He created a circle of movement from the most extrovert to the most introvert, and placed his twelve healers around the circle. Mimulus, for example, reflected a state of fear 'of those who quietly and secretly bear their dread',[8] but also it reflects a great tenacity in the face of difficulties. It is often found clinging to a stone on a river bank, and reflects that it is 'possible to live happily amongst dangers and find freedom through the acceptance of our situation'.[9] Unable to tolerate pollution, mimulus is fast disappearing from the streams of the British countryside. Impatiens, thought to be the first remedy discovered by Dr. Bach, and possibly reflecting his own constitutional type, reflects the tendency to be quick thinking and impatient, irritable and tense. Intolerant of others who are slow, the impatiens type will often prefer to work alone. Bach noted that although the plant has very rapid growth and its seed pods disperse with a violent action, the flower is delicate. In its positive aspect it grants a state of gentleness and forgiveness.

Bach went on to discover what he called the twelve healers, which address the twelve constitutional states of imbalance, the twelve soul types. Later he discovered the seven helpers, which are not type remedies, but relate to specific situations an individual may be passing through. Olive, for example may be used when the energy is very low, wild oat when the thread of the life lesson has been lost. Dr. Bach felt that he had completed his task, but he was led to discover another nineteen remedies, usually referred to as the 'second nineteen' which are used for more transitional emotional states. The twelve healers and the seven helpers are made by laying flowers in a bowl of spring water and allowing the sun to shine through the flowers into the water. The water is then imprinted with the essence of the flower. The second nineteen, sometimes called the boilers, are prepared in quite a different way, being heated by fire from below. These second nineteen have a different function in that they enable learning through experience of life.

Dr. Bach suggests that illness has the power of 'bringing back the personality to the divine will of the soul'. He suggested that all life is connected, that in nature there is no separation. Any action against this basic unity of life he saw as the most severe of our human errors. Bach reasoned that if we could learn these soul lessons there would be no more need of illness, or 'the severe lessons of suffering'.[10] Fear, he suggested, is the most divisive of the emotions, leading to withdrawal and self-obsession, and is the cause of many illnesses. Boredom he maintained as another main cause. In the true spirit of his time, he suggested that if we all take full interest in the world about us, learning from every possible situation in life, there would be no room for boredom, no place for fear.

Since his death, the Bach Flower remedies have gained reputation and popularity. He gave freely of his knowledge and suggested that we all follow his instructions and make our own flower remedies. During the past 15 years there has been a proliferation of flower essences, the best known being the California Essences and the Australian Bush Essences. Many other flowers have been tried and tested and given their therapeutic assignation. But the system of Dr. Bach still has much to offer. He felt that his thirty-eight remedies covered all that was necessary for us to move forward into health. By working with the energies of plants, as Dr. Bach suggests, maybe we can begin to understand the constitutional patterns of belief and behaviour which prevent us from becoming truly human.

In the presence of the way of nature, disease has no power. [11]

Chinese medicine

Chinese medicine is based in a Taoist philosophy which sees mankind as living between the energies of heaven and earth, *yin* and *yang*. *Yang* describes the attributes of heaven, *yin* the attributes of earth. Between heaven and earth is a constant flow of energy/information which is called *qi*. Classical Chinese medicine is rooted in the belief that in order to be healthy one must live in accordance with the laws of nature and with what is natural. Living according to the laws of nature and following one's own true nature is following the *tao*. Chinese medicine stresses the importance of the cycles of nature, and bases its 'laws of the five elements' on an observation of the energetic changes in nature throughout the four seasons. Spring is seen as the time of birth, growth and expansion, summer as the time of openness and fruition. Autumn is a time of decline and letting go, winter a time of withdrawal, separation and death. These cycles are the cycles of life, and if life is to be maintained these cycles must be honoured. Too much expansion and there will be imbalance. Too much withdrawal and there will also be imbalance. *Yang* expresses the outward energetic movements of spring and summer, *yin* the inward, nourishing aspects of autumn and winter.

Within Chinese medicine, the interaction of *yin* and *yang*, the two poles of opposition create the dynamic tension of life. *Yin* and *yang* represent the polar opposites of pairs such as hot and cold, hard and soft, assertive and yielding, neither one being possible without its energetic counterpart. It is the pattern of this dynamic tension, the movement between *yin* and *yang*, which is suggested by *qi*, and it is this pattern which is affected by acupuncture treatment. Chinese energy medicine includes massage techniques—the most common being *tui na* in China and *shiatsu* in Japan—and exercise, particularly *qi gong* (literally working with *qi*) and *tai chi*. *Shiatsu* balances *yin* and *yang* by using specific techniques and recognizing which parts of the body are full and which are empty. *Tai chi* attempts to balance *yin* and *yang* with both strong and yielding postures. Oriental forms of exercise differ from Western forms in that they stress not only movement or posture, but also breath, awareness and intention. Intention (*yi*) is considered to be an integral part of the healing process. It is by motivating intent that change is able to take place. Intention is what unites the biology with personal destiny, and puts the individual in touch with the *tao*, the way of nature. Western science, however, has attempted to explain its mechanisms a little differently.

In 1971, an American journalist observed a surgical operation in Beijing with acupuncture as the only means of anaesthesia. His observations were reported in the New York Times and stimulated much interest by the scientific and medical communities in the mechanisms of acupuncture. Early research suggested a purely neurological effect (the 'gate-control' theory), whereas later research proposed the involvement of chemical mechanisms such as the release of endorphins and other naturally occurring opiates within the central nervous system. Because of a proven link with endorphin release, acupuncture gained a certain respect amongst the medical and scientific communities for the treatment of pain. Further research has shown that various other 'neurotransmitters' are affected by acupuncture treatment, and that different chemicals may be activated or deactivated according to the type of stimulation, usually electrical, given to the needle. This later research has shown that the effects of acupuncture on the treatment of pain are more complex than was first expected: what could have been a simple explanation was seen to be simplistic.

While this research may have some validity in the attempt to understand its painkilling effects, pain control is a very small and recent development within the whole spectrum of Chinese medicine. Pain control is just one aspect of the body's complex informational system, and maybe the release of endorphins is just one of the many chemical mechanisms that acupuncture can trigger in the body. The research of Dr. Candace Pert (described in the second chapter) may have much to offer in understanding the mechanisms of acupuncture. The energy/information systems of the body proposed by 'energy medicine' may be found to have a close relationship to the movement of neuropeptides and the implied relationship between the nervous, endocrine and immune systems.

Homoeopathy

Within CAM, certain disciplines address the 'patterns of information' directly, rather than concentrating on the unbalanced part. Acupuncture addresses the *qi*, and homoeopathy the 'vital force'. Although its medicines are drawn from the natural world and include animal, vegetable and mineral products, the effect of homoeopathy is not directly physical or biochemical. The preparation of homoeopathic medicines involves the continual dilution and trituration (shaking or vibrating) until no single molecule of the original substance remains. A homoeopathic remedy contains the 'energetic imprint' of the original material, and the 'higher' the potency of the remedy, the more dilute the substance. According to William Tiller of Stamford University:

> Conventional allopathic medicine deals directly with the chemical and structural components of the physical body. It can be classed as an

objective medicine and thus has much direct laboratory evidence to support its physiochemical hypothesis. Homeopathic medicine, on the other hand, deals indirectly with the chemistry and structure of the body by dealing with substance and energies at the next, more subtle level. It must be classed as a subjective medicine at this time because it deals with energy that can be strongly perturbed by the mental and emotional activity of individuals, and in part because there has not been any diagnostic equipment to support the homeopathic physician.

He concludes:

. . . our future treatments will proceed towards the development of techniques and treatments that utilize successively finer energies.[12]

Disillusioned with a medicine which seemed to cause as much suffering as it relieved, homoeopathy was discovered by Samuel Hahnemannn at the end of the 17th century. A prominent German physician, he turned his back on a successful career and began translating and writing. Hahnemannn was a chemist and a linguist, and he embarked on an extensive study of the *materia medica*, translating texts from the Greek, Arabic and Hebrew. Chinchona, or Peruvian bark, had recently been introduced to Europe as a cure for malaria, interested to discover more about its effects, he began experimenting with small doses and noted his symptoms. After a few days he contracted symptoms similar to those of malaria. This was the first of many such 'provings' of medicinal substances and poisons, and he soon felt confident that a substance which is used to treat symptoms in a sick person, produces those same symptoms in a healthy person. He experimented for seven years 'proving' various substances, until he felt that he had a sufficiently wide range of medicines to begin treating patients again. He had some success, but was still concerned about the ill-effects that many of the substances, they cured the main symptoms, but caused other 'side effects'. He began to try out smaller and smaller doses in order to find safer ways of treating. Hahnemannn discovered that smaller doses of a substance could still provide an effect, but his most astonishing discovery was that by shaking the diluted substance it became more 'potent'. This led to a radical departure from the mainstream of medicine, and caused Hahnemannn's medicine to be ridiculed by the doctors of the time. 'Potentization' recognizes that as a remedy becomes more dilute physically it becomes more active energetically. Remedies are produced today in the same way that Hahnemannn described, with a procedure of serial dilution and succussion. According to Hahnemannn it is the succussing or shaking of the remedy which allows the energetic imprint of the substance to be imbued on the carrier, which is generally water. We have seen that the chemical structure of water is such that it creates an electromagnetic field. The molecules of water are able to bond with many substances and the water will change its molecular structure depending on which element it is bonding with. The nature of water may prove to be important in the ability for a remedy to hold the information of a substance even though no actual molecules of the substance remain.

Homoeopathy suggests that remedies have healing potential, but that the power to heal is within the individual not within the remedy. If the medicine has a resonance with the patient it will stimulate self-healing. The practice of homoeopathy therefore is dependent on matching the remedy to the patient. The closer the match, the more effective the treatment. Hahnemann described this self-healing mechanism as the 'vital force'. J. T. Kent, the 19th century homoeopath, describes the vital force as 'formative intelligence' that not only operates every material substance, but it is the cause of cooperation of all things.[13]

Homoeopathy is widely used in the treatment of animals; for example it has proved to be effective for cows with mastitis. It has become a favoured system of health care amongst farmers who rear their cattle using organic methods. Similarly for children, the remedies are easy to take and childhood illnesses can be treated naturally and safely.

Despite its wide acceptance, particularly within the UK where it has always had royal patronage, the mechanisms of homoeopathy remain a mystery to science. Madeleine Ennis, professor of immunopharmacology at Queen's University, Belfast, recently headed a study which involved four separate research centres. Each centre was sent one phial of pure water and another of water containing histamine at a homoeopathic dilution. They were not told which tube was which. All four centres found that the dilute solutions inhibited histamine release from basophils, just like histamine itself.[14] Ennis said that if her results were real we may have to rewrite physics and chemistry. But Peter Fisher, director of research at the Royal Homoeopathic Hospital in London suggests that it may be all in the changes to the structure of water. Somehow information is stored in water, and the act of preparing a homoeopathic remedy imprints this information on the water. Ordinary untreated water has no structure. Professor Ennis reluctantly concluded:

> Despite my fundamental reservations against the science of homoeopathy, the results compel me to suspend my disbelief and start searching for a rational explanation for our findings.

The web of healing

We can see from that each of the therapies discussed above has its own perspective on health, its own perspective of healing. Holism may be seen by different therapists in different ways. To some it is looking at the whole body, and seeing all bodily symptoms as interconnected, a sore throat may be connected to a bladder problem, a sexual problem to lower backache. To others it is the inter-relationship of bodily symptoms with emotional blockages which inform their diagnosis and treatment. Someone holding back emotions will often hold their breath. The result may be asthma, but the therapist may need to encourage the patient to address the emotional causes before they are able to experience relief. In homoeopathy the more symptoms—physical, mental and emotional—that fit the remedy picture, the more effective the treatment. Similarly, in Chinese medicine an attempt is made to create a pathology picture which includes all symptoms, not simply to add them all together, but to weave a 'pattern of disharmony' which will provide a simple yet effective treatment. An osteopath will look at the structural alignment and understand an underlying problem of organic function. No one therapy is more holistic than another—the holistic nature of treatment depends on the ability of the individual practitioner to see the multi-dimensional layers of the individual problem, and on the ability of the patient to respond and to embrace change.

If the therapist remains stuck in the role of practitioner as expert, the patient as passive receiver of treatment, the patient may benefit from the treatment, but will not necessarily be empowered by the encounter. If on the other hand the practitioner is able to share knowledge, to give the patient a means to understand his or her problem, and to provide suggestions for self-help, the patient will be able to regain some control over his or her life. But knowledge exchange is not only verbal. Inherent within an Alexander Technique session, an acupuncture treatment, and a homoeopathic remedy is the idea that the body can learn more healthy patterns of behaviour. In whatever way is congruent with their particular mode of treatment, the practitioner can aid the patient towards self-healing.

Patients and practitioners can become partners in health. Using a system of cooperation not domination, doctors will be able to help their patients to understand the disease process and become part of their own cure. The present system is one of extreme disempowerment, where victim consciousness is both endorsed and encouraged. And as we have seen from the work of both Deepak Chopra and Carl Simonton, attitude effects disease. Rather than handing over their personal power to the expert, CAM encourages the participation of the patient in the healing process.

The work of general practitioner Norman Shealy with medical psychic Carolyn Myss has suggested that certain negative attitudes have a specific relationship to illness. Negative belief systems and the lack of ability to use the power of choice to directly affect our lives are seen to have a major impact on health. According to Myss and Shealy, 'decision making powers should be seen as a fundamental survival skill for life'.[15] As patients we need to ask more questions, empower our decision making by being more informed about our health. As practitioners we need to empower patients to take on responsibility. The original meaning of a therapist is an attendant, or 'one who watches over'. The patient does the healing. The practitioner facilitates the process.

Chapter Four

Sustainable Health

During the second half of the twentieth century Complementary and Alternative Medicine struggled to gain acceptance and credibility; practitioners dealt not only with their patients' doubts but also their own. Some of the more established therapies attempted to fit in with the current scientific perspective of orthodox medicine in order to become more respectable. Doctors took up short courses in homoeopathy, or used acupuncture for the treatment of pain. Nurses began to use essential oils to relax their patients. The whole field of CAM has gradually matured, and now is the time for practitioners and patients to share knowledge and experience, the time to begin serious cross-discipline dialogues in an attempt to understand more about the healing process, and to interact on a more meaningful level with orthodox medicine in order to begin to create a new model of health and disease. We need to integrate the different schools of thought into a new conceptual framework.

Complementary and Alternative Medical practitioners need to talk to conventional medical doctors, not trying to fit in to the current system, but instructing on holism. With less demand to provide proof that CAM works, researchers will be able to spend more time on discovering how it works, because it is by discovering how these therapies work that we will gain more understanding of the body/mind and the healing process. CAM has much to offer conventional medicine in its understanding of the body as a whole. By working together we can attempt to create new partnerships for health.

Any real change to our health care system must be a two-way process, of enlightenment within the profession and on-going education of the public. Rather than simply blaming our failing health care system, we can all begin to create change by taking more responsibility for our own health. Over the past 50 years we have given away the control of our health to professionals. Simple health care must become de-professionalized. We need to regain our common sense, regain our trust in our bodies and re-learn the simple skills of cooking nutritious food and taking regular exercise. Teaching children about health is the most important step towards a future healthy society. Every school child could learn how to use natural remedies to deal with cold and flu symptoms. This simple step would alleviate GP overload and provide some relief to a common problem for which orthodox medicine has no answers.

We need to develop a clearer view of the connections between our own health, the health of the community and that of the environment. In *The Triple Health Challenge*, Michael Renner draws a global picture of health by outlining the environment, human and economic factors that effect the health of the world's population:

> The health of human societies and the natural environment is strongly related to how robust they are in the face of adverse developments.[1]

We are all becoming aware that current farming methods undermine health: both our individual health and the health of the environment. We are beginning to understand that human health and environmental health are one. We are part of nature, and the past two hundred years of the domination of science over nature has served to cut us off from the roots of our health. The prerequisites for life on earth are pure air, clean water and nutritious food.

Any lasting change in health care will come from three main areas:

- personal responsibility
- collective responsibility
- education

Personal Responsibility

Lifestyle choice affects health. Smoking kills three million people a year, and is the largest single preventable cause of death.[2] As well as cigarettes we also enjoy alcohol, junk food, watching TV, driving cars and working too hard. As we exercise less and consume more sugar and fats, one in six people are considered to be overweight, and this is a major contributing factor of chronic diseases such as stroke, heart disease, cancer and diabetes.

Eco-economist Hazel Henderson suggests that one of the main problems facing the world today is that we live in an age of 'do as I say, not as I do'. In answer to a question about the health of physicians, she suggested that in the past a healer was expected to be in touch with health in the same way that a priest is supposed to be in touch with God. In discussion with Fritjof Capra, she suggested that if we all began to 'walk our talk' then not only would we be personally empowered but some real changes may take place. She likened the problem of health care with the environmental movement, where she suggests that everyone was happy to talk about environmental problems, but how many people were actually doing something about it? They may belong to the Sierra Club, she suggests, but how many sort their garbage and economize on electric power? She goes on:

> But there has been a whole evolution of consciousness within the environmental movement. It is becoming imperative that once you begin to make these connections, you can no longer speak with forked tongues. You can no longer go round describing what everyone should do without trying to be a model yourself. So you end up not pointing the way but being the way, and if you can't be the way, you just have to get out of the ballgame because you become such a charlatan.[3]

There are many reasons why we do not take responsibility for our health. In the UK, we have lived the past fifty years under a state-organized health system which has proved to be a double edged sword. It has provided health care for all, but at what cost? The result has been a demoralized and obedient public who no longer felt qualified to take the smallest decisions in the field of health care. A public wide open to the propaganda of the drug companies and insurance brokers spinning their tales of fear and alarm.

As individuals we have tended to accept without thinking various practices that have become so familiar in Western society. For many years it has been the practice of dentists to use amalgam fillings or more recently to apply a protective plastic coating to help prevent tooth decay in children. Likewise, the majority of us have been ready to allow the mains drinking water to be treated with fluoride in order to prevent tooth decay. Women have gratefully accepted their hormonal balance to be altered to prevent pregnancy or to remove the symptoms of menopause. Fear encourages us to vaccinate our children against diseases, and we accept x-rays, the use of MRI scans and ultrasonic diagnostic machinery.

Whilst we do not necessarily suggest that we should shun all recent technological or biochemical medical developments, we must become more aware of what we allow to be done to us in the name of health care. We can be more responsible for our own health by being more aware of the choices we are making.

Recently an even more sinister trend has arisen. Drug companies play not only on our fears but also on our competitive nature and job insecurity. Recent advertising campaigns for cold and flu relief medication placed mostly on transport systems, suggest that if you take time off to recover from your cold, you may lose your job. So why not take the medication and carry on working? It may damage your immune system in the long term, but at least you will not be seen to be slacking. This clever marketing strategy exploits the current pattern of behaviour which rates overwork above health. It is fashionable not only for doctors but for alternative health care professionals too, to show that they are busy, stressed and overworked. Of course, the health system is under stress and many doctors do not have the choice, but alternative practitioners are generally self-employed, and can chose to take time out. But a sense of responsibility towards their clients, or possibly a need to pay the mortgage (or own a second car?) will often win over personal health care. In modern society our self-worth is often tied up with how busy we are, how much we are able to achieve. Our self-worth does not seem to be augmented by being healthy, but rather by showing others just how stressed and overworked we are.

Many people do not want to take responsibility for their own health because it means changing their lifestyle and habits. There is a general lack of incentive in a society where there is an absence of role models that provide positive health image. It may be argued that the popularity of sport may provide such models for the young, but modern sport and the popularity of the gym culture may be more about building strength and physique than promoting health. And to many teenagers it is still more fun to be rebellious, as may be seen in the increase of smoking amongst teenage girls. As we grow older, the lack of responsibility for health may grow from a sense of powerlessness in the face of a health care system which has not promoted understanding or self-responsibility. Our society has suffered from a lack of education about health, coupled with an overload of information on diet, vitamins and exercise regimes. But change has already begun to take place, and the move towards alternative systems of health care and the increase in self-medication with natural remedies is a sign that a shift of consciousness has begun. According to Caroline Myss:

> The rapid growth and development of the holistic health field indicates that our needs are changing in fundamental ways and that the model of traditional medicine and health care cannot adequately meet these needs. Fundamental change means that movement is taking place at the very core of human nature itself. What is the nature of this evolutionary change now taking place? A transformation is occurring in terms of how the concept of responsibility is understood and then applied to every aspect of one's life.[4]

The public are, in increasing numbers, demonstrating their desire for a more people-centred approach to health treatment. There is clearly a demand for a more holistic approach to treating disease, as demonstrated by the recent report in the *New Scientist* (May 2001) where it claims that in 1999, 28.3% of the population used complementary and alternative therapies in England. In the same year £450 million was spent on CAM in the UK. The average patient is far more informed than ever before due to information access via the internet and various patient support groups which promote understanding and information to the public. This can make patients not only take a greater role in their own health, but also give them the opportunity to view prospective treatments and make the choices which they prefer.

Collective responsibility

In a recent talk given by Sir Christopher Paine at the Royal Society of Arts in association with the Royal Society of Medicine, he pointed out that:

> It seems doubtful whether our progressively more centralized NHS, with its national targets, its guidelines, protocols and other top-down instruments of regulation, is going to foster what society wants from health care.[5]

In the Schumacher Briefing *The Ecology of Health*, Robin Stott has made a number of recommendations in linking causes of ill health to a range of proposed solutions. These are measures that can be implemented at a local level and the progress monitored by the local community. He sets out a vision for a new health system by involving local people in health management decisions. He suggests that we adopt a system of primary care groups which will in time create networks with other organizations and initiatives that relate to health. He emphasizes the need to put individual health at the centre of local planning suggesting that:

> The new role of health professionals is in advocacy and education, so that all can understand the wider health implications of initiative . . . health workers will give leadership through advocacy and example. . . . When people's values are incorporated into our health systems, we will be well on the way to gaining health—enhancing social and environmental change.[6]

Decisions need to be made on a human scale, and interactions must be carried out within the local community. Recent initiatives in the USA, Europe and other parts of the world signify trends towards public involvement in the health decisions that we are now facing. Ethics committees, which are outlined in Andrew Weil's *Roots of Healing*,[7] now include a panel of citizens to discuss individual cases where decisions of an ethical nature are needed. He states that in 1982 only 1% of the hospitals had ethics committees but by 1993 this had increased to more than 60%. These are ways to encourage a partnership approach to health and to ensure that medical decisions are made for the benefit of the patient. However, a real commitment to health education is essential if these public-involving initiatives are to work. There will be greater motivation and the system will work more effectively.

But these initiatives could be taken further so that the public are not only involved in the decision-making processes of the system itself, but also in their own healing process. This could be greatly helped, as Robin Stott rightly pointed out, if the public were more informed about the environmental and political causes of ill-health, but there could also be initiatives to educate and inform the public so that they are able to take more responsibility for their own health. With the introduction of natural therapies into the public health system, it would be possible to demonstrate that through using simple and effective natural remedies it is possible to treat many of the small and minor illnesses oneself. There could be an exchange of knowledge, with the individual gaining confidence to deal with their own problems by learning from other people in the community. Furthermore, by using natural remedies or growing herbs, it is possible to learn their properties, thus regaining much of our lost traditions and home remedies. Learning to heal oneself is both empowering and fulfilling.

Community health centres could become the providers of health information for all ages and all members of society. They could become the communication link and focus within every borough of the country. They could work directly with the hospitals or main care services and make a start in shifting the balance away from medically-based, research-driven drug treatments and towards health care. They could bring real health care back into the community, but with a holistic approach. Information could be accessed by the use of data bases and on-site resources; the individual would be able to make an informed health decision based on information and guidance.

These centres can offer advice on alternatives that will lead to healthier living. Our health includes the food that we eat, the air that we breathe, and the way that we use our bodies. Centres could provide classes in nutrition, exercise, breathing techniques, as well as to provide information on environmental factors. The public is now demanding to know more about the connections between the quality of our environment and our health. Whether they are concerned about the increasing incidents of agricultural disaster or about public health warnings concerning the safety of beaches, they are making these links: the health of the environment effects our own well-being.

It is questionable whether we have paid sufficient attention to the quality of food. Over the past sixty years we have produced food at the lowest possible cost through industrialized farming and processing. These methods are now leading to outbreaks of 'mad cow' disease and to the recent uncontrollable foot and mouth epidemic. Together with the widely used practices of prescribing antibiotics and hormone treatments to animals, there are inevitable links to be drawn between modern farming methods and individual health. The food that we eat should be nutritious and safe. Governments could encourage the production of organic food, recently shown in the latest Soil Association report to provide more nutritional value than conventional food:

> The evidence supports the hypothesis that organically grown crops are significantly different in terms of food safety, nutritional content and nutritional value from those produced by non-organic farming.[8]

Greater vigilance should be encouraged in the use of food additives. The food additives aspartame (marketed as Nutrasweet, Equal and

Spoonful) and MSG (monosodium glutamates), for example, have been linked with allergies and behavioural problems and therefore have been banned from all organic foods.[9]

As we begin to understand more about nature, maybe we will begin to see that the health of our bodies and the health of the land are related. We apply chemical medicines to the body in a similar way that we apply herbicides or pesticides to the land. In the same way that we no longer feel able to take the time to learn about our illnesses and to overcome them in a natural way, we are not willing to weed or learn through good agricultural practise how to avoid pests, and to naturally enhance the productivity of the land. Our bodies and our land are locked into a race of productivity, with no time to rest and no time to lay fallow.

In the 21st century we are beginning to see the true cost of environmental clean up. Together with the pollutants from the fertilizers, pesticides and herbicides used in agriculture, the impact from industry is still increasing. Waste, including nitrates, petrochemicals and chlorine, is threatening the quality of our water. Many illnesses can be traced back to polluted air, water and food, and it is the responsibility of the government to ensure good practice within industry. The cost of health should not be paid by the individual taxpayer whilst the polluters of industry and farming benefit. There is now a need to encourage good environmental practice within business and the public sector, and to promote sustainable agriculture.

Health spending is a major cost for the UK Government. The NH budget is £59 billion annually and there is always enormous pressure to increase funding. Physical and mental health problems also bring major costs to other government departments, such as social security, and to the economy as a whole through lost working days. As long as government health policy focuses on treating symptoms as opposed to improving health these costs are expected to increase. In comparison only £3 billion is spent directly on UK agriculture each year by DEFRA (Department for Environment, Food and Rural Affairs) under the common agricultural policy. And only a very small fraction of this is targeted at encouraging and developing organic farming.[10]

Changes are starting to emerge in the world of business. Aware of the potential environmental and health issues at stake, industry is beginning to look at its social and environmental responsibilities as well as its financial responsibilities to its shareholders. Through the work of organizations such as Forum for the Future, SustainAbility and the Social Venture Network, there is a move to change practice and to gain stakeholder approval. It will inevitably make financial sense in the long term to reduce the use of non-renewable energy and other resources. Again, greater government encouragement could be given to these initiatives. It may be expensive to initiate and create the necessary changes in practice, but this would undoubtedly result in a cleaner, healthier environment. Social health implications in these new business initiatives should also be recognized. A business that focuses on the welfare of its workforce will result in healthier, happier employees. Some companies now provide aromatherapy massage to help reduce stress or include sports facilities to encourage exercise.

The role of the government is sharply brought into focus when we examine the question of the pharmaceutical companies. Until we break the hold of the drug industry there can be no real change within the health care system. Dinyar Godrej states in the *New Internationalist*:

> The roots of drug abuse in Western medicine lie in the profession of the apothecary, who could not legally charge patients for health advice, only for pills and potions. . . . it was the advent of 'miracle drugs'— antibiotics—from 1930 to 1950 that led to the marriage between doctors and the drug industry and thence to the widespread susceptibility of the general population to pill-popping.[11]

We must question the drug companies' motives. To whose benefit are these sales, and to what extent do they really benefit the health of the individual or the environment? With the indiscriminate and over-prescribing of antibiotics there is a danger of developing mutated bacteria and hence creating new diseases. A further danger is that overuse of antibiotics causes damage to the friendly bacteria, particularly the intestinal flora which form an important part of our natural defence system, hence weakening the body against disease. We need to examine the extent of the relationship we have to the drug companies as they seek to spread their markets. If increased use lessens the effectiveness and demands further use or creates dependency, surely comparisons can be drawn with the illegal drug market, where the producer pushes up the need of the consumer and profits from it. Here we have a government-sanctioned situation which holds an unhealthy power by the mere size and influence of the industry.

G. Cannon suggests that an estimated $9 billion is wasted every year because of the irrational use of antibiotics.[12] Michael Renner makes the point that at least half of all antibiotics used in human medicine are prescribed unnecessarily.[13] The influence of the pharmaceutical companies does not stop with the drive to sell medicines. They are also in the business of creating food additives, agricultural chemicals and carrying out research in genetic engineering. The cycle of creating a demand to promote sales continues, as we have seen with the creation of markets for hormone replacement therapy. With a higher annual turnover than some of the countries they supply, drug companies can be more powerful than the countries themselves. We must always be careful to decide whether their work is really of value, and perhaps recommend that the UK government separates its interests from their activities. MCA, the drug-regulating quango supported by the DHSS, has on its board existing directors of pharmaceutical companies. We must remind ourselves that they are first and foremost beholden to their shareholders.

The major drug companies are now developing 'over the counter' natural medicines and are promoting the need for standardization of herbs. It is not in their interest to acknowledge that we can become healthy by using natural remedies, many of which you can grow in your own garden. The customer does have a right to feel confident that a natural product conforms to a professional standard, but maybe we should ask ourselves whether we would prefer an organically grown, naturally produced product rather than one whose chemical components have been adjusted to a pharmaceutical formula. There is a danger that the drug companies will change the holistic nature of natural medicine into a chemicalized version that is really not that much different from the drugs that they already sell. This process of 'standardization' is being carried out in the name of research and progress, but it continues to maintain the power of the professional and the drug companies. Unfortunately, one of the major forces against the implementation of the use of natural medicines must be the drug companies.

Education

We need to create a school environment that encourages children to become individuals, not simply training them to function in roles set by the current economic demands. Children are naturally inquisitive and eager to learn. They are also creative, and with responsible, wise education they can develop into people who will be able to live healthier, more equitable lives. They will be able to contribute to the health of society by being wise parents themselves as much as by being a computer technician or environmental engineer. Healthy children need to learn that they are creative beings, by developing a sense of responsibility for their community, by learning how to recover from setbacks and above all by being able to experience their own value. We create all the time. Everything we do is an act of creation because we choose everything that we do and how we do it. It is more to do with the way you approach your life. In *The Creation of Health*, Caroline Myss suggests:

> In our very beings, we know that we need to learn as children in order to become effective adults, and part of that inner knowledge is that we know we need to learn how to be responsible for what we create as well as to learn what it means to create responsibly. We need to know how to communicate on our own behalf. We need to know how to handle the consequences of our actions. . . . Self-expression and creativity are crucial to health—and not just physical health. The creation of a healthy life—as well as body—requires that a person maintain dominion over his or her life.[14]

She goes on to say that violation of our creative being does not prevent us from being creative but that 'negative outlets' are discovered. Children need encouragement to express who they are and what they feel. They need to feel valued, and we can help this process by providing them with the opportunity to follow their interests and develop skills. We can give them clear guidelines to help them make choices, teaching children in a way that does not destroy their natural interest. We all need to feel that we are members of the community that we live in, part of a family or neighbourhood or social group. Children develop ways of interacting with others and grow in confidence to trust their judgement. Being able to trust their own intuition develops their sense of self-esteem. This helps them to negotiate their way through relationships, starting at school and continuing during the rest of their lives. To be able to grow within a caring community helps us grow with a sense of security, and we are able to develop a sense of respect for others. We will not undermine our own health and the health of others by making work more important than our friends or our families. This can be reinforced in schools by supporting the teachers to adopt a more caring role and fostering respect and self-worth amongst the pupils.

We can gauge our health by how well we can recover from illness and our ability to resist disease. We can teach children ways in which to encourage resistance to disease by looking after the body and eating well. And although it could be argued that poverty may be an obstacle in providing an adequate diet, it is much more expensive to live on a diet of junk food than on simple, natural and nutritious food. Within schools, we could be setting an example, serving organic, fresh, healthy and tasty food at school instead of the standard school meal that is centrally produced and encourages unhealthy eating habits. Healthy schools initiatives are being developed in many boroughs in the UK, and although this is encouraging it does not venture into discovering the real implications of how our lifestyles impact on health. Parents and teachers can help children recover from physical, emotional and mental setbacks. Fostering awareness of health and the issues surrounding health at an early age will enable children to eventually choose to be healthy rather than unconsciously undermining their vitality and immunity.

The curriculum could become more relevant and more practical, particularly in areas where there is increasing disaffection from boredom and truancy in schools. At this stage, children and young adults can learn about the connections between human action, society and the world as a system in itself. We can teach the principles of sustainability and make the connections with creating a healthy world. These ideas which can be communicated through the educational system will need to be incorporated into the fabric of the teacher training courses. Food for Health courses could be included, as well as academic and exam-oriented studies. They can be used as part of a vital part of building their knowledge of the world. For many years compulsory sports activities were part of the basic requirements for the school curriculum, but this regime in more recent years has been overshadowed by the need for academic attainments. However, once again, particularly with the initiative of the lottery funding for sports, schools are recognizing the value of exercise in school. It would be preferable to encourage the development of fitness and strength rather than using sports as a way of encouraging competition and rivalry. We can adopt the practice of traditional schools of the Far East and teach martial arts to promote discipline, relaxation and the development of skills, as well as physical strength and fitness. Circus skills, dance and outdoor-challenge activities are ways of developing skilful movement and fitness in the body.

There are recent initiatives to include entrepreneurial skills into schools, such as 'Business in Education Schemes' which have been set up to give children a way in to the reality of working. They can gain real experience in business and this idea could develop to become a mainstream activity in secondary education. Children can learn that social and environmentally responsible practice is more likely to generate sustainable services and products. It will help children understand the effects of research, design and manufacture on their health and the health of society and the environment. There is a need to develop institutional changes towards sustainability. In 'Futures 32' Roy emphasizes:

> . . . the need for developing innovative ways of thinking about the services that usually underlie the products that people want, and how these might be provided sustainably, rather than the characteristics of the products/services themselves.[15]

This is a challenge we can encourage children to work with, whether it is learning about energy alternatives for the future or the ways to create clothing free from the toxic cocktails in many modern fabrics. Although children can be involved in this innovative work, the real challenge is to help them think beyond the present boundaries and in ways that are not restricted by 'physical thinking'. Becoming practically involved in the search for healthier alternatives can be a highly creative process, demonstrating the importance of taking responsibility for the decisions we make. This could be the cornerstone of education.

In order to create a more holistic health care system, there must be a willingness on all sides for dialogue and change. As much as orthodox medical professionals need to accept that the holistic approach has its place within medicine, so do alternative and complementary practitioners need to be willing to dialogue with the medical profession and within itself.

Nic Rowley in *Basic Clinical Science* suggests:

> A fragmented approach to medical education persists because of difficulties in knowing where to start when faced with the huge volume of material now available for study and may account for the fragmented approach to the human condition manifested in some practitioners.[16]

A change can be developed during the training of the medical professionals by integrating natural medicines into their curriculum in order to demonstrate a holistic approach. We need to encourage a participatory approach to their training, so that they learn to listen to patients and work with them through the healing process.

Natural medicines such as acupuncture are already being used in some hospitals, but rather than challenging orthodox medicine by introducing the concept of energy medicine into mainstream, it tends to be used merely for pain control—a version of acupuncture which has been approved as acceptable by medical science. Currently doctors and physiotherapists learn acupuncture in short courses which do not allow for the holistic philosophy of Chinese medicine. But we would suggest that if alternative therapies are introduced into the orthodox medical system, they should be studied within the context of their philosophy on health. Only then would students develop an understanding of holism and the true potential of natural remedies.

The shift from a treatment-based approach to a care-based system can only start with changing the emphasis in the medical schools. We would suggest that existing natural medicine practitioners can support this process. The teachers of the various therapies can open channels of communication with the orthodox medical world and become involved in the philosophical part of the training as well as teaching about the traditional remedies. Natural practitioners must guard against their own prejudice and remember that their role in the healing process is to facilitate the patient towards health.

Holistic approaches to health and healing are vital for us all. Through using natural medicines it is possible to reconnect to our own power to heal, and we can all be involved in this process. We cannot sustain our health without addressing what is needed throughout the interconnected systems of our lives; our selves as individuals, our physical health, our psychological health, our relationships with our families, our communities and our environment. In regaining the roots of our health, we may learn to be better stewards of the earth as well as of ourselves.

References

Chapter 1
1. Lea, Bill, quoted in *Cultural and Spiritual Values of Biodiversity*, UNEP, Intermediate Technology Publications, 1999.
2. Berlin, E.A. and B., *A General Overview of Mayan Ethnomedicine.*
3. Ibid.
4. Malidoma Patrice Some, *Of Water and the Spirit*, Penguin Arcana, New York 1994.
5. Hillman, James, *The Force of Character and the Lashing Life*, Ballantine, 1999.
6. Quoted in Greer, Germaine, *The Change*, Hamish Hamilton, London 1991.
7. Greer, Germaine, *The Change*, Hamish Hamilton, London 1991.
8. Quoted in Greer, Germaine, *The Change*, Hamish Hamilton, London 1991.
9. Greer, Germaine, *The Change*, Hamish Hamilton, London 1991.
10. Chopra, Deepak, *Perfect Health*, Bantam Books, 1990.
11. Heindal, Max, *The Vital Body*, The Rosicrucian Fellowship, 1950
12. Tisserand, Robert, *The Art of Aromatherapy*, C. W. Daniel, 1977
13. Hamlyn, Edward, *The Healing Art of Homoeopathy: The Organon of Samuel Hahnemann*, Beaconsfield, 1979.
14. Kaptchuk, Ted, and Croucher, Michael, *The Healing Arts*, BBC Publications, 1986.

Chapter 2
1. George Engels, quoted in *The Turning Point*, Fritjof Capra; Flamingo 1977
2. Planck M. *The Philosophy of Physics*, New York, 1936.
3. Zukov, Gary, *The Dancing Wu Li Masters*, Rider, 1979.
4. Ibid.
5. Oschman, James, *Energy Medicine: the scientific basis*, Churchill Livingstone 2000.
6. Ibid.
7. Oschman, James, *The Natural Science of Healing*, research papers, 1986.

8. Firebrace, Peter and Hill, Sandra, *A Guide to Acupuncture*, Constable, 1994.
9. Gerber, Richard, *Vibrational Medicine*, Bear and Co, 1988.
10. Capra, Fritjof, *Uncommon Wisdom*, Flamingo 1988.
11. Bateson, Gregory, *Mind and Nature*, Dutton 1979.
12. Quoted in Oschman, James, *The Natural Science of Healing*, research papers, 1986.
13. Goodwin, Brian, *How the Leopard Changed its Spots*, 1994.
14. Ibid.
15. Tiller, William, 'Illness as a Biofeedback Mechanism for the Transformation of Man', research paper, Stanford University, 1979.
16. Silverman, Julian, *The Musculo-skeletal Research Project*, Aspen Research Institute, 1981.
17. Quoted in Capra, Fritjof, *The Turning Point*, Flamingo, 1977.
18. *European Journal of Oriental Medicine*, Vol.3 No.4, Winter 2000.
19. Pert, Candace, *Molecules of Emotion*, Simon and Schuster, 1997.
20. Chopra, Deepak, *Quantum Healing*, Bantam Books, 1989.
21. Capra, Fritjof, *Uncommon Wisdom*, Flamingo, 1988.

Chapter 3
1. *New Scientist*, May 2001.
2. Kaptchuk, Ted, and Croucher, Michael, *The Healing Arts*, BBC Publications, 1986.
3. McCarthy, Margot (ed.), *Natural Therapies*, Thorsons, 1994.
4. *New Scientist*, May 2001.
5. Chevallier, Andrew, *Encyclopedia of Medicinal Plants*, Dorling Kindersley, 1996.
6. Kaptchuk, Ted, and Croucher, Michael, *The Healing Arts*, BBC Publications; 1986.
7. NYR Foundation Course in Natural Medicines.
8. Chancellor, Philip, *Handbook of the Bach Flower Remedies*, C. W. Daniel, 1971.
9. Barnard, Julian and Martine, *The Healing Herbs of Edward Bach*, Bach Educational Programme, 1988.
10. Bach, Edward, *Heal Thyself*.
11. Bach, Edward, *The Seven Helpers*.

12. Introduction to Vithoulkas, George, *The Science of Homoeopathy*, Grove Press, 1980.
13. Vithoulkas, George, *The Science of Homoeopathy*, Grove Press, 1980.
14. *New Scientist*, May 2001.
15. Myss, Caroline and Shealy, Norman, *The Creation of Health*, Bantam, 1988.

Chapter 4

1. Renner, Michael, *Vital Signs 2001: The Trends that are Shaping our Future*, Worldwatch Institute, 2001.
2. WHO, *World Health Report*, 1995.
3. Capra, Fritjof, *Uncommon Wisdom*, Flamingo, 1988.
4. Myss, Caroline and Shealy, Norman, *The Creation of Health*, Bantam, 1988.
5. *RSA Journal*, 1st April 2001.
6. Stott, Robin, *The Ecology of Health*, Schumacher Briefing No. 5, 1999.
7. Weil, Andrew, *Roots of Healing: the new medicine*, Hay House, 1997.
8. Soil Association, *Organic Farming, Food Quality and Human Health*, Soil Association, 2001.
9. Ibid.
10. Ibid.
11. *New Internationalist*, Issue 272, February 2001.
12. Cannon, G., *Superbug: Nature's Revenge*, Virgin Books, 1995.
13. Renner, Michael, *Vital Signs 2001: The Trends that are Shaping our Future*, Worldwatch Institute, 2001.
14. Myss, Caroline and Shealy, Norman, *The Creation of Health*, Bantam, 1988.
15. Roy, 'Beyond Single Vision', *Futures* 32.
16. Rowley, Nic, *Basic Clinical Science: Describing a Rose with a Ruler*, Hodder and Stoughton, 1994.

SCHUMACHER BRIEFINGS

The Schumacher Briefings are carefully researched, clearly written booklets on key aspects of sustainable development, published approximately three times a year. They offer readers:

• background information and an overview of the issue concerned
• an understanding of the state of play in the UK and elsewhere
• best practice examples of relevance for the issue under discussion
• an overview of policy implications and implementation.

The first Briefings are as follows:

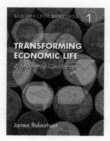

No 1: Transforming Economic Life: A Millennial Challenge by James Robertson
Chapters include Transforming the System; A Common Pattern; Sharing the Value of Common Resources; Money and Finance; and The Global Economy. Published with the New Economics Foundation.

No 2: Creating Sustainable Cities by Herbert Girardet.
Shows how cities can dramatically reduce their consumption of resources and energy, and at the same time greatly improve the quality of life of their citizens. Chapters include Urban Sustainability, Cities and their Ecological Footprint, The Metabolism of Cities, Prospects for Urban Farming, Smart Cities and Urban Best Practice.

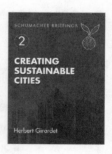

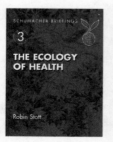

No 3: The Ecology of Health by Robin Stott.
Concerned with how environmental conditions affect the state of our health; how through new processes of participation we can regain control of what affects our health, and the kinds of policies that are needed to ensure good health for ourselves and our families.

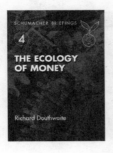

No 4: The Ecology of Money
by Richard Douthwaite

Explains why money has different effects according to its origins and purposes. Was it created to make profits for a commercial bank, or issued by government as a form of taxation? Or was it created by users themselves purely to facilitate their trade? This Briefing shows that it will be impossible to build a just and sustainable world until money creation is democratized.

No 5: Contraction & Convergence: The Global Solution to Climate Change by Aubrey Meyer

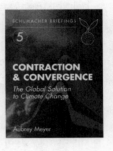

The C&C framework, which has been pioneered and advocated by the Global Commons Institute at the United Nations over the past decade, is based on the thesis of 'Equity and Survival'. It seeks to ensure future prosperity and choice by applying the global rationale of precaution, equity and efficiency in that order.

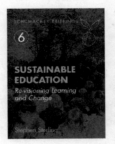

No 6: Sustainable Education: Revisioning Learning & Change by Stephen Sterling.

Education is largely behind—rather than ahead of—other fields in developing new thinking and practice in response to the challenge of sustainability. The fundamental tasks are to • critique the prevailing educational and learning paradigm, which has become increasingly mechanistic and managerial • develop an ecologically informed education paradigm based on humanistic and sustainability values, systems thinking and the implications of complexity theory. An outline is given of a transformed education that can lead to transformative learning.

Future Briefings will deal with issues such as food and farming, globalization, local development, environmental ethics, energy policy, alternatives to genetic engineering and green technology. The Briefings are published by Green Books on behalf of the Schumacher Society. To take out a subscription, or for further details, please contact the Schumacher Society office (see next page).

THE SCHUMACHER SOCIETY
Promoting Human-Scale Sustainable Development

The Society was founded in 1978 after the death of economist and philosopher E. F. Schumacher, author of seminal books such as *Small is Beautiful*, *Good Work* and *A Guide for the Perplexed*. His sought to explain that the gigantism of modern economic and technological systems diminishes the well-being of individuals and communities, and the health of nature. His works has significantly influenced the thinking of our time.

The aims of the Schumacher Society are to:

• help assure that ecological issues are approached, and solutions devised, as if people matter, emphasizing appropriate scale in human affairs;

• emphasize that humanity can't do things in isolation. Long-term thinking and action, and connectedness to other life forms, are crucial;

• stress holistic values, and the importance of a profound understanding of the subtle human qualities that transcend our material existence.

At the heart of the Society's work are the Schumacher Lectures, held in Bristol every year since 1978, and now also in Liverpool and Manchester. Our distinguished speakers, from all over the world, have included Amory Lovins, Herman Daly, Petra Kelly, Jonathon Porritt, James Lovelock, Wangari Maathai, Matthew Fox, Ivan Illich, Fritjof Capra, Arne Naess, Maneka Gandhi, James Robertson and Vandana Shiva.

Tangible expressions of our efforts over the last 20 years are: the Schumacher Lectures; Resurgence Magazine; Green Books publishing house; Schumacher College at Dartington, and the Small School at Hartland, Devon. The Society, a non-profit making company, is based in Bristol and London. We receive charitable donations through the Environmental Research Association in Hartland, Devon. Schumacher Society Members receive:

• a free lecture ticket for either Bristol, Liverpool or Manchester
• the Schumacher Newsletter
• the catalogue of the Schumacher Book Service
• information about Schumacher College Courses
• a list of other members in your area, on application

The Schumacher Society, The CREATE Environment Centre,
Smeaton Road, Bristol BS1 6XN Tel/Fax: 0117 903 1081
<schumacher@gn.apc.org> <www.schumacher.org.uk>